I0569793

Welcome back:

A TBI recovery story from Provider to Patient

Mandi Dickey, FNP-BC, MSN, RN
Minneapolis, MN
brainwellnessnp@gmail.com
https://brainwellnesssolutions.com/

Brain Wellness Solutions © 2024
ISBN: 979-8-9908612-0-6

Acknowledgements

This book would not have been possible without the encouragement and help from my husband, Don, my biological and nonbiological children, my friends Krissy, Amanda, and Elise, and my entire treatment team that helped me get to where I am now.

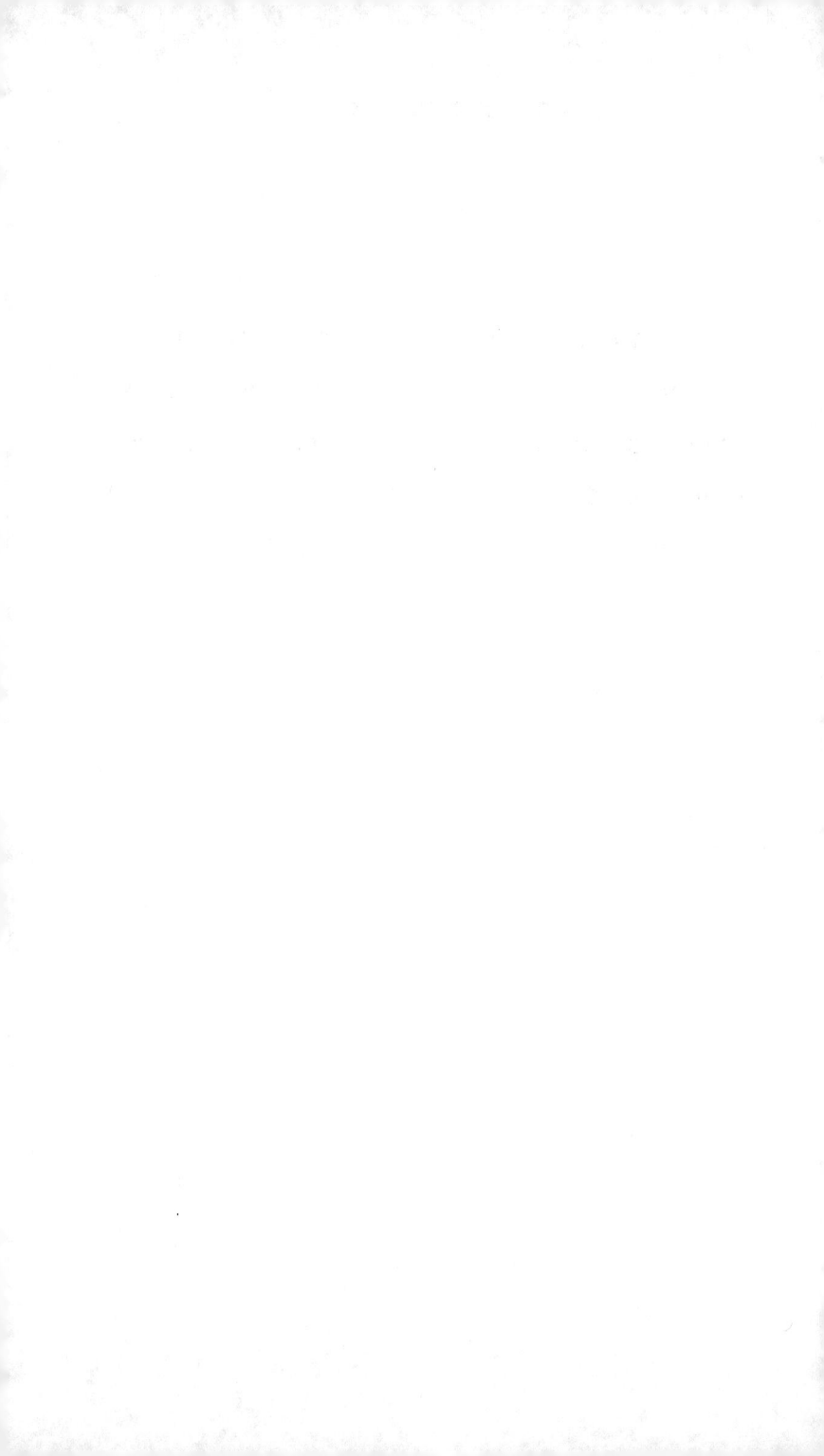

Introduction

After nearly 6 months of struggles, we rode in the car and I talked my child's ear off. He finally chuckled, smirked, looked at me and said, "Welcome back". But let's back up a bit to find out what I had to come back from…

I was always a go-getter, working multiple jobs, raising kids while going to school to further my degrees. I initially went to college thinking I wanted to be a music major, but it clearly wasn't meant to be as I kept running into snags in my education plan. I took a break from college, found a local course to become a nursing assistant and fell in love with healthcare. I decided nursing was my new passion, and all the doors started opening up for me.

I began by getting my associate degree in nursing, went straight into my bachelor's degree while working as a nurse, then straight to graduate school for my master's degree in nursing. I used my master's degree to work in management for a while, then switched to teaching the future of nursing as faculty in a nursing program. After a few years of teaching, I realized I really missed having my own patients and wanted to be back at the bedside fulltime, so I went back to school for my nurse practitioner certificate (this was a post-master's certificate, accelerated program - yay!).

Essentially all of my healthcare experience was in neurosciences to some aspect. I spent a few months on a general medical/surgical floor before transferring to the neurology floor as a nursing assistant while in nursing school. I stayed there as a nurse after graduating with my associate degree, then spent time in the ICU for a while (always including neuro patients) as both a floor nurse and in management before moving on to teaching. Even as a professor, I had the privilege of creating a 1-credit elective course for neuroscience-inclined students.

When I went back to school for my nurse practitioner (NP) certificate, I knew exactly what my goal was - to work as a neuro NP. And that is exactly where I landed. I spent 11 years in neurology before looking to expand my knowledge into the other areas of neuroscience and ultimately, I took a new job in a surgical group where I would care for brain and spine patients.

Not gonna lie, my life was getting pretty much perfect at this point. As I went through all these magnificent years in neuro, some not-so-magnificent things were happening in the rest of my life. I had two tough marriages with difficult divorces and three kids between the two marriages - the youngest had just been diagnosed with autism the year prior after years and years of struggling with behavior issues and various therapy attempts without success. I had finally found my perfect life partner and had just gotten engaged, the kids were doing great in school (including my youngest who was FINALLY excited to go to school and was doing phenomenal off all of his medications), and I had just switched to this exciting new job.

Then the unthinkable happened...we were in a car accident...and I felt like I had been hit by a bus, but it was an SUV. And that's where this story really begins...

1

In the blink of headlights

I remember the day like it was yesterday, but the days between get pretty fuzzy. I was at my highest high - I was in orientation for my new job and thought the day was going to be spent in the clinic as was listed on my schedule, but the doctor that I was shadowing had surgery on his schedule for the afternoon, and I got to tag along. I was only a month into my job, and I couldn't touch anything because I was still just 'shadowing' (learning without the hands-on aspect, literally).

The surgery staff got me gowned up and tied the arms of the gown behind my back, 'mummy style' as they said, so I wouldn't accidentally touch anything. I got to stand right next to the surgeon, however, and watch the entire procedure! I got his permission to ask questions as he went along, because I wanted to soak up every aspect of the experience. I got to be in the OR for a brain surgery, something I had wanted to see since I got into healthcare 24 years ago.

When I got home, I talked my new fiancé's ear off about the surgery - I was still on cloud nine from the experience. His birthday was a few days away and his birthday present had arrived early (a new tool to work on our compound bows). He was excitedly playing with the tool, seeing how it worked, while he chuckled at me as I talked nonstop. I waited for him to get done playing with his new birthday present so we could go to dinner, but it was getting late, so I reminded him one last time we should get going before the restaurant closed. He reluctantly left his new tool, and we hopped in our vehicle.

I kept talking the whole ride, which normally lasts about 10 minutes - I was just so excited about the surgery! We were at the last intersection before the restaurant, and I could see the restaurant on the corner. The light turned green, or so we thought - we would later learn through traffic camera footage that only the straight light turned green - our turn light was still red. There was one car coming from the other direction on the highway; they had their headlights on, and you can see for half a mile at least on this stretch of the road, however they made no attempt to stop or swerve or slow down as we were going through the intersection.

There was no honking of the horn, no squealing of the tires; they just crashed into our car at full speed, slicing off the front end right in front of the wheel on my side of the vehicle. As I later learned, after hitting us, they continued moving through the intersection and stopped against the traffic light post - they were moving at some impressive speed.

The last thing I got out was "Babe!" as I saw the headlights coming at our car. Then everything was like slow motion but fast at the same time. When Don (my fiancé) realized the other car was not stopping, he quickly did what he could to try to minimize the impact from the accident - he turned the wheel as far as he could to try to match the angle of the other car so it wasn't a direct hit to the side of our vehicle. I felt the crash of the vehicle (a midsize SUV) hitting us and the shifting of our large SUV.

Amid everything else moving so fast, this is the moment that time slowed down for me. It felt like one of those slow-motion moments in a movie, as I could feel my head violently bouncing to the left and to the right until our vehicle came to a stop. The airbags throughout the vehicle deployed, sending fluff and dust into the air - it became difficult to see inside the vehicle.

My phone and wallet had been tucked between my knees as we drove (so I could talk with my hands as I always do), and they were thrown to the floor by the impact. Once everything stopped moving, I heard Don ask "Babe, are you ok?" and I realized I was hyperventilating, repeating "Oh my God, oh my God". I couldn't get out any other words in my panic.

After a few moments, Don pushed his door open and fought through the airbags to get out. He came around my side of the car and forced the door open to check on me. As my phone was thrown to the floor, apparently it engaged the emergency feature and 911 was automatically dialed. Don was able to reach my phone for me as we were connected with a dispatcher.

My left knee swelled up instantly and I started to feel pain. I noted scratches down my right shoulder and arm that were bleeding - we would later identify that these scratches were from the airbags and suspected that my knee was impacted by my phone and wallet that had been tucked there. Don went to check on the other driver and came back right away once he could tell the driver was ok - he was already out of his vehicle and walking around. It seemed, at the moment, that the only one injured was me.

When officers got there, they checked on us and asked a few brief questions. The ambulance crew came over with a stretcher and had me pivot from the car to the stretcher. My knee was swollen and painful, so no one wanted to take any chances of having me walk on my own. Then they wheeled me around the front of the vehicle and into the back of the ambulance. This was the moment of truth for me - I started feeling panicky when I saw that the

5

front of our vehicle was completely missing from just in front of the tire. Headlights were hanging by their cords, I could barely see into the vehicle because of all the airbags obstructing the view. Don was talking with the police as I rolled by him.

I couldn't feel all of my pains yet, but my coping mechanism has always been humor, so I tried joking with the paramedics. I got an IV placed but told them I didn't need anything for pain yet (adrenaline was still blocking the pain at this point). They put a neck brace on me just in case there was cervical spine injury as I was just starting to feel some discomfort in my neck, and we waited for Don to come into the ambulance to ride with me to the hospital. They asked him if he wanted to be evaluated, too - he said 'sure' but didn't really feel any symptoms yet at this point. They got both of us logged on their tablet and got vital signs on both of us.

The ride to the hospital was fairly uneventful. I got an ice pack for my knee but wanted to hold off on anything for pain because I wanted to be able to give the ER doctor an accurate evaluation. Don called his best friend to come meet us at the ER, because we were going to need a ride home eventually. Once we got to the ER, we found out the call had apparently been placed incorrectly - I wasn't listed as the right level of "trauma" so they transferred me from the stretcher to a wheelchair and parked me in the waiting room. I remember thinking this was a bit off.

Some time later I was taken back to a triage room. I was examined briefly for visible injuries and imaging was ordered, including scans of my head, neck, shoulder, and knee. After the imaging was completed, I was wheeled back to the waiting room again to wait for results. At this point I still had received nothing for pain, and I was sitting in a wheelchair with a c-collar on my neck and ice pack on my knee. A most bizarre experience, indeed. Everything was starting to throb - my left knee, my right shoulder, my low back, my neck, my head...

Our friend sat with us in the waiting room. I don't remember all of the conversations, but I remember we waited a long time. Eventually, our friend took Don home to get our other car while we continued to wait on results and for the ER doctor to finally see me. While they were gone, I was taken back to see the ER doctor. Imaging results had all come back - I had no clear fractures, no obvious head trauma, just some soft tissue changes in all areas of pain. I had a brief evaluation by the ER doctor, and I then waited again for another employee to come finish everything with me.

My knee was bandaged up and I was given crutches, though I asked how that was going to work since my right shoulder was also swollen and painful. I had more questions than answers at this point. I never did get anything for pain and my IV was taken out. I had a muscle relaxant ordered for discharge (but it was the middle of the night so I wouldn't be able to get it until later), and I was again wheeled out to the waiting room to wait for Don to get back. He opted not to be seen since he was feeling stiff all over but generally fine and didn't want to make me wait any longer to get home.

Don wheeled me to the car and got me and my crutches loaded up. I started panicking about the drive home, not really excited to be back in a vehicle already. We had to get home, though. We joked a bit (we both have the same twisted coping mechanism) and drove through a Taco Bell drive thru because it was the only thing open, and we never got to our dinner.

Don had to get up and go to work in the morning (which was now only a few hours away) because there were no other supervisors on the schedule. He was stiff and had a headache, but he pushed through as he always does. I slept in…because pain kicked in. When I woke up, I took note of all of my bruises, which seemed to have multiplied while I slept. I took some ibuprofen for my head and went back to bed. I thought I'd only be out of work for a day or two - I thought I just needed some rest.

We were supposed to have Don's birthday party that night with our friends, but I had sent a message to the group from the ER that we were going to postpone because we were in an accident. This was the smart idea of our friend with us in the ER - I couldn't think of what to do about it. She was

9

very wise in recommending we postpone - I had no idea how much pain I was going to be in. I was supposed to go to work (it was now Friday), but I had also messaged my boss and supervisors from the ER that I was going to need a day of rest. They were very understanding and wished me well.

2

Whispers of trauma

The accident happened on a Thursday evening. On Saturday we decided to go look for a new car. We knew our vehicle was totaled and I was going to need something to get to work the next week (or so we thought). We drove to a few dealerships and looked around - the vehicle we totaled was a Toyota Highlander, one of the top three safest SUVs on the market because of all the airbags and safety features. We decided we wanted to get another Highlander because of the safety rating, and because the vehicle had saved our lives. We ideally wanted to find a hybrid, but we were having difficulty finding a used one.

At the second dealership we stopped at, we carefully looked down the row of Highlanders in the sales ramp then turned around and found the twin to the vehicle we had just totaled. This one had the interior color Don had initially wanted when we got our other Highlander the year prior, so we thought it was meant to be and took it home.

I didn't drive the Highlander home that day - I drove my Ford, but I still ugly cried the whole way home driving any car. I was scared shitless being back in a car again (pardon my French). This made no sense to me, however, because I was the passenger in the accident - why in the world was I scared to *drive* a car? I called one of my best friends to "be with me" while I drove home. Don drove to a friend's house where he was working on a project, so he wouldn't be home for a few hours. I didn't want to be alone, but I was crying too hard to talk much. I realized after this that I was going to need a couple more days before I could go back to work, because I had no idea how in the world I was going to drive myself there in this state.

3

All hands on deck

At this point, I reached out to a neurologist friend (whom I had worked with at my last job), whom I had also seen for my migraines in the past. I told him about my accident and asked to be evaluated for concussion. He was glad to squeeze me in that week, so I would be off work until I saw him and got further recommendations. I was still hoping things would be fine and I would be back to work possibly by the end of the week (though I still wasn't sure how I was going to drive myself there).

At my appointment, my neurologist friend Identified that I had significant visual and balance troubles. I apparently wasn't in a cognitive state where I could identify these issues myself. I thought I felt "off" but I couldn't really describe how. He referred me to an eye doctor for further evaluation of my visual difficulties and physical therapy (PT) to work on my balance.

Having worked in neurology for as long as I had, I have connections all over the place (which came in very handy on multiple occasions). I had gotten a recommendation from a friend/former colleague for an eye doctor who specialized in post-concussion evaluations who happened to be practicing in my metro area. I had mentioned this to my neurologist, and he was all for it. I called and made an appointment for the first available, the following week. So now I would be off work until I saw the eye doctor and got further recommendations. I was honestly ok not going back to work yet at this point, as I was sleeping half the day away every day, yet still completely exhausted, everything hurt, and my head was now screaming at me on a regular basis.

The following week, I went to my eye doctor appointment, but it wasn't exactly the easy appointment I had hoped for. The eye clinic had two locations and while I thought I had asked for the one closest to me, I had gotten scheduled at the first available, which was twice the drive. When I got to the clinic where I thought I was supposed to check in, they informed me of my error, and this threw me completely for a loop. I started crying and left the clinic. In my head, I needed this evaluation so I could get back to work, and I had no idea how I was going to get it rescheduled in time to get evaluated and get back to work the next week. The clinic called me while I sat outside crying and offered that the eye doctor could still see me that day at the other location if I could head straight there. I managed to calm myself enough to drive and got myself to the farther away clinic.

I didn't exactly have a simple exam and I didn't get the ok to go back to work. I could only tell him that I didn't clearly see two objects, but I also didn't clearly see one single object in my vision - everything just seemed…blurry. Through a multitude of testing, he identified that I actually had significant diplopia (double vision) and prescribed prism glasses for correction. I would have one pair with my prescription correction so I could work on the computer and one pair without my reading prescription to wear the rest of the time. The hope with these glasses was that they would correct the diplopia enough while I waited to get into occupational therapy (OT) for vision therapy, ultimately so I could get back to work hopefully sooner than later.

I ordered my sets of prism glasses, though I admit this also was a bit difficult, because when I looked in the mirror to see how they looked on me I didn't see one single clear image and had no idea how the frames actually looked on my face. It would take nearly two weeks for my prism glasses to come in, and I now needed to wait to get back to work until these were obtained to help me see the computer, and had to wait to go back to work also until after starting OT to get a better timeframe for returning to work related to my visual difficulties and the necessity of being able to work on the computer for most of my day. The appointments were endless, as were the delays it seemed.

4

Fractured sight

In healthcare these days, everything is on the computer - I would need to be able to review my patients' charts, review their imaging, write orders and notes, and all of this was done on the computer. When I saw my eye doctor for the first time, I could only tolerate 30 minutes on a screen before my headache severely increased. Apparently, this was because of the work it took to focus my eyes in order to read the screen. I thought things just seemed blurry - I had no idea there was a bigger issue.

My first hint at visual problems (before I had gotten to the eye doctor) was one week after the accident. We had a field day for the firearm safety class I was teaching with my dad - I had to shoot a shotgun as an example for the students and on this day could only hit one clay pigeon - the previous year when we held this class, I couldn't miss the clay pigeons (even shooting left-handed due to an elbow injury a few months prior). I thought it was just fatigue, but in hindsight it was likely the diplopia.

As I mentioned previously, in the eye doctor's office he had me do all sorts of evaluations. He had me sitting upright, leaning back, and attempting to read things from various angles. Ten years ago, I had lens implants in both eyes due to severe myopia (nearsightedness) that I've had since I was born, so because of the severity of trauma from the accident, he also checked the location of my lens implants to make sure they hadn't been knocked out of place. From what he could tell, they weren't.

In addition, he had me do specific testing for diplopia. There were so many dots on the screen in front of me - apparently there were just supposed to be a few. I saw dots in a variety of different colors - they moved to the left and right or up and down, depending on the kind of prism the doctor put in front of my eyes. I didn't think it was clearly one object I was looking at, but it also wasn't clearly two…until I did the testing. Then it became *clear* that I truly did have double vision. I left that first appointment so nauseated from all the prisms being taken on and off and going back and forth between one and two objects in front of me.

Waiting for the prism glasses seemed to take ages. They told me it would take two weeks for them to be made and available for me, and they were nearly spot on. I couldn't use my regular prescription glasses because it didn't seem to correct even my prescriptive issue, not to mention the diplopia. Without the prisms, I could tolerate about 30 minutes on the computer before focusing on the screen caused a significant headache and fatigue.

When I got my computer prisms (which arrived first), I could tolerate up to an hour on the computer, but still got a significant headache from focusing on the screen so much, so I couldn't do it very often. The regular prisms seemed to make things clearer when I was driving, but didn't seem to help with anything else, so to be honest I only wore them when I was driving. I called the eye clinic again and tried to make an appointment to re-check my vision because the prisms didn't seem to help much.

When it came time for the appointment, however, the clinic called me to cancel - the eye doctor wanted me to get vision therapy first, because he thought ultimately that was going to help more than the prisms. So again, I had to wait for the next appointment to happen.

When I got to my first OT appointment for vision therapy, she did more testing and identified that not only did I have significant diplopia, but I also had reduced peripheral vision and near complete inability to see nearly anything around me if I was focusing on an object in front of me (this felt essentially like tunnel vision).

I also had reduced speed on computer testing in which I had to identify the directions of arrows that appeared on the screen. I had to press the corresponding arrow on the computer keyboard when I saw the arrow on the screen. We did this with both eyes open then with each eye individually. While my results were technically 'within normal limits' it was at the very slow end of normal, and for my age, my OT expected me to be much faster. So, we decided to meet regularly, and I got exercises to work on at home in between appointments. I wouldn't be going back to work yet because I needed to increase my visual tolerance. Looking back, this was likely one of the first exams to correspond with my cognitive issues that would be identified much later.

After doing vision therapy for a while and wearing my prism glasses, I went to a follow up exam with the eye doctor. Since it wasn't such an emergent exam, he had more time to dig deeper into my chart and noted my previous prescription (prior to the lens implants). I used to say I was blind as a bat, but my oldest child corrected me years ago and said bats weren't as blind as me because they could use echolocation, which I clearly could not. My left eye prior to my surgery was about -12.5 diopters and my right eye around -22 diopters. I don't remember the exact numbers currently, but these are approximately correct.

I didn't just have the lens implants in both eyes, I also had LASIK surgery on the right eye for further correction, because my eyesight was so poor. After both procedures, I was reading off the

20/20 line for the first time in my life. It was exhilarating. But it only lasted 3 years before I had to have some sort of correction again. You see, I had, and still have, what is known as progressive myopia. It is progressive deterioration of my near vision (nearsightedness, or myopia), which will continue throughout my life. The surgery didn't correct the myopia, it just set me back to a new baseline because I was wearing contacts and glasses together in order to see prior to surgery - neither would correct my vision enough alone anymore.

The diagnosis I wasn't aware of with this severe myopia I had was 'refractive amblyopia'. My eye doctor described this as similar to regular amblyopia, which is more commonly known as "lazy eye". Whereas with regular amblyopia one eye has muscle weakness that causes the eyes not to track together, with refractive amblyopia there is muscle weakness due to the severe discrepancy in prescriptions between the two eyes that essentially causes the patient to have monocular vision (only the stronger eye actually provides useful information to the brain).

He suspected that since I didn't have correction for that as a child, that my brain was essentially only getting information from my left eye for most of my life. Now that my brain was injured, it was trying to get information from both eyes, so we essentially 'woke the sleeping bear' - we woke up the eye that wasn't supposed to be giving information to my brain…and now it was giving all sorts of information. This would cause problems with healing.

Because of this new realization, he gave me a patch to wear over my weak right eye to try to decrease my symptoms so we could retrain my eyes to work together - essentially do the treatment for the amblyopia that I didn't receive earlier in life. With the patch on, I could tolerate an hour on the computer without increasing my headache, but as soon as I took the patch off, the headache would come back with a vengeance.

The next thing we tried was 'binasal taping' on my prism glasses to reduce strain on the right eye and try to retrain my peripheral vision. This required literally putting a piece of tape on the inner part of the lens on both eyes (i.e., 'binasal') to prevent my eyes from trying to converge on the object. Honestly, my eyes didn't want to converge anyway - I also was experiencing what was called 'convergence insufficiency'. Normally when we look at an object, our eyes 'converge' or track together to send the same image to the brain. My eyes didn't want to connect, so this was part of the reason I was seeing double - they weren't cooperating to send a single object to my brain.

The taping didn't do the trick. Taping almost seemed to put more focus on the right eye instead of reducing the strain and my headaches were getting worse. So, then we added a colored dot to the center of the lens on the right side, to try to again decrease the focus on the right eye while keeping my peripheral vision activated. This, however, seemed to reduce my peripheral vision further and I felt like I was going to run into walls, and I couldn't wear the dot while driving.

The vision in my right eye seemed to be getting worse - my vision seemed really fuzzy when I tried to look just out of my right eye, almost like I had never had the LASIK done. After a week or so, we transitioned away from the dot and then the tape on the non-computer glasses due to my further vision issues. My OT and eye doctor were communicating regularly to discuss my treatment plan and relay their recommendations to me.

My OT was doing well, but this was now getting outside of her experience, and she admitted she might not be the right person to continue working with me on these exercises. Then came a referral to a more specific vision therapy center under the direct guidance of an optometrist, as my problem seemed to be a rare issue given my previous eye difficulties compounding the new difficulties from the concussion.

Months later I would gain the ability to put my thoughts into imagery, so I was finally able to make an image that explained how my vision felt: literally like everything was blurry and dark.

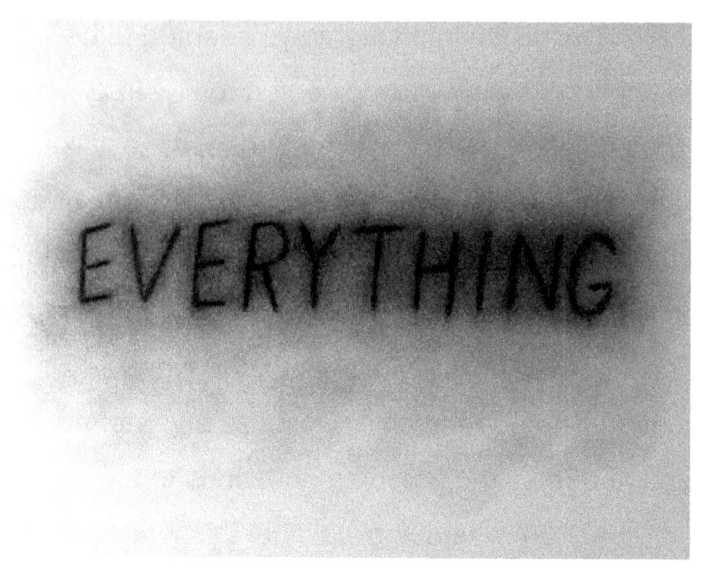

While waiting to get in for the more advanced vision therapy, I noticed my prisms weren't helping as much anymore and suspected I had some changes in my eyes, so I made another follow up appointment with the eye doctor. We again did a bunch of testing and did a lot of on and off with prisms. I had started some new therapies (which will be discussed later in the book) and had noticed some improvements with both PT and OT. Here was another improvement - I no longer seemed to need the horizontal prisms! We took a moment to celebrate this win, because wins seemed few and far between for me. Then we had to discuss the things that didn't improve, and actually seemed to worsen.

I still needed the vertical prisms, and ultimately, he suspected I would need some sort of prism long term, i.e., permanently. Even prior to the car accident, I noted difficulty navigating stairs when I walked down them and had a history of losing my footing. Apparently when I look down, my eyes deviate, which likely is causing my unsteadiness when walking down stairs. For this reason, he suggested that whenever my eyes stabilize, he will likely need to add a prism to the bottom of my lenses to prevent this sensation when looking down.

As previously discussed, I had really bad eyesight prior to the accident, leading to lens implants to give me a new baseline for correction. I was told when I got the implants that I would be at a higher risk for development of cataracts, and a year prior to the accident, my regular eye doctor had estimated I would need cataract surgery in 5 years or so because I was, indeed, developing cataracts. With the new therapies I had been receiving, I was more cognitively aware of what was going on, including being more aware of my deficits. I was not feeling as foggy and could identify my symptoms more readily. Therefore, I was readily aware of the fact that my vision wasn't as clear, and when the prisms weren't working as well, I could tell.

Through the testing we did, my eye doctor identified that my prescription needs had changed - I had a higher prescription than at previous visits. He suspected this was because my cataracts had visually progressed. He now suspected I would not be making that 5-year mark for cataract surgery - it likely will be much sooner. This made me wonder if the car accident sped up the formation of my cataracts.

Historically, it was believed that only trauma to the eyes would lead to increased risk of cataract formation, but a recent study published in October 2023 evaluated military service members who had trauma to the eyes compared to those with no trauma to the eyes, and there was still an increased risk of cataract formation if there was no direct trauma to the eyes[1]. So, one could presume that my

TBI did, indeed, increase the rate of my cataract formation.

In addition to this, I was now able to identify that even when I closed one eye (more specifically my left eye) I would still see things blurry and somewhat double. My eye doctor noted that this usually comes from something wrong inside the eye itself...and inside the eye was my lens implant. He again shone bright lights into my eyes to try to visualize the implants, but he could not rule out the fact that the implants may have moved ever so slightly, or be slightly curved, so that I was no longer seeing clearly through them. The only correction to this would be surgery, and he suggested that this would be taken care of whenever I need to have my cataracts corrected. So, I have this to look forward to, I guess.

My new prism glasses were ordered and only took a week to receive this time. After obtaining the new lenses, I also was able to get in for my first appointment with the new OT to work on more advanced vision therapy. My first assignment? Playing with a tennis ball. Time to work on some hand-eye coordination as well as peripheral vision. Next came work on visually tracking letters on a sheet of paper - working both on visual perception and processing. Eight months since the accident and my peripheral vision and visual processing were still major problems.

5

The maze of forgetfulness

A week after the accident, Don and his daughter and I were out running errands in the afternoon and stopped for lunch. I was getting tired, and my headache was kicking in after driving around and having to use my brain to think about things. We went to a Vietnamese restaurant for pho - Don had never tried it before but was open to trying something new. I got Thai tea, which one of my best friends had introduced me to a few years ago. Don had never tried Thai tea before and I told him he should really try it because it was amazing, and his daughter agreed. Apparently, he tried it, and a few minutes later I again was telling him he really needed to try it because it was amazing. They both looked at me like I was crazy and said he just did...I still don't remember him trying the tea.

Looking back through text messages, I also found a message I had sent to Don that I had gone to the pharmacy in that first week after the accident to pick up my medications, but forgot the name of the medications I needed to refill (I only have a few prescriptions, so there's not much to remember) and had to make multiple trips back and forth to the pharmacy to get the names of the medications correct. I was clearly frustrated.

That's about the time it became clear to me that I wasn't remembering things well. I still didn't remember fully all the events in the ER the night of the accident; I really just remember the highlights. In the weeks after the accident, I didn't remember who I had told about the accident and who I hadn't. When I did talk to people, I repeated stories to them multiple times; my kids started giggling when I would do that with them. I was constantly forgetting what I was doing and where I was going. I went to the wrong location for appointments on multiple occasions (the clinics had multiple locations and sometimes I was scheduled at a different one if there was not an opening at my primary clinic).

Essentially, if something wasn't on my calendar or to-do list, it didn't get done.

Examples of things I'd forget:

a. Names of people (didn't matter if I'd just met them or knew them for a long time)

b. Birthdays and anniversaries, even if they were on my calendar and I had just looked at them

c. Appointments, or locations of appointments

d. Food - in the oven, on the stove, on the counter (if they needed to be refrigerated), in the car (if I had just gone grocery shopping) or on a couple occasions at the end of the conveyor (after paying for them and forgetting to bag them at the store)

e. Whether the dogs had been fed

f. What day of the week it was

g. Take my medications/supplements

h. Refill my pill box when it ran out

i. Refill prescriptions when they ran out

j. Pick up my medication refills

k.   Eat breakfast or lunch (dinner was a given
        with the family, but the other meals were hit
        or miss)

l.   Conversations, right after they were had

m.   Directions on how to take new medications

n.   Exercises from therapies - what to do, how to
        do them, how often to do them (some were
        daily, and some were every other day)

o.   Passwords I had just changed

p.   What happened on the TV show we just
        watched

q.   Whether bills were paid yet or not

r.   Answers to medical questions when friends
        would message me for advice

s.   Doses of supplements I'd recommend to
        people for migraine (which I used to
        recommend on a nearly daily basis at work
        and even wrote a dang book about it)

t.   The location of organs or nerve patterns in
        the body (something I learned in anatomy 24
        years prior and have stressed the importance
        of knowing to my students and new
        employees ever since)

u.   How to sign my name without having to focus on each individual letter when signing a document…

It has been so frustrating not being able to remember things as well as I'd like. I feel like my medical knowledge is nearly completely gone, or at least nearly completely inaccessible. If I get distracted while talking, I often still immediately forget what I was talking about. Until recently, if I struggled to come up with a word in a sentence, I would lose my train of thought in the conversation. If I had a conversation about one thing related to the accident, I couldn't remember who I spoke to about it and often forget to tell other people. I had a couple of good friends I had reached out to along the way, and if I talked to them about something, unfortunately I often forgot to tell Don, so he was sometimes inadvertently left out of the loop. I didn't realize how big of a problem it was initially.

Much later in the process of recovery, I would learn to start keeping a spreadsheet with dates of appointments and when I made phone calls so that I would hopefully be able to stay on top of things better. I was dropping the ball on a lot of things, and not keeping Don in the loop on these things caused problems. When I created the spreadsheet, I looked back at text messages and even notes from my care providers to recall what had been happening up to the point of starting the spreadsheet. I had months pass and couldn't remember what all had happened during that time.

We all have times when we forget something we usually know. In typical everyday life, if you can't remember a detail about something, you can "Google" it. You can get online and use some sort of search engine to find the information you're looking for. We can't do that with the memories that are stored in our brains, though. There's no search bar to find exactly what we're looking for.

Often enough, we can't retrieve a memory we are looking for, but most of us just shrug it off and move on. People that have some form of dementia or other brain issues may struggle more than others. Truthfully, there are days I have *felt* like a dementia patient - I would repeat the same information over and over and ask the same questions over and over…but I was not the one realizing this - my family was, and less so my friends (only because I didn't talk to them as often as my family).

My biggest concern was that I just haven't been able to access the basic information I want to. I still often can't remember what the term is that I want to say, and sometimes can't come up with an explanation of it enough to help others understand what I am trying to say. I feel like my main search engine is out of order - it just doesn't want to work. When my brain finally did start functioning better and I was able to put this thought into an image, it felt to me like being on a computer where you get an error message when you're trying to find something.

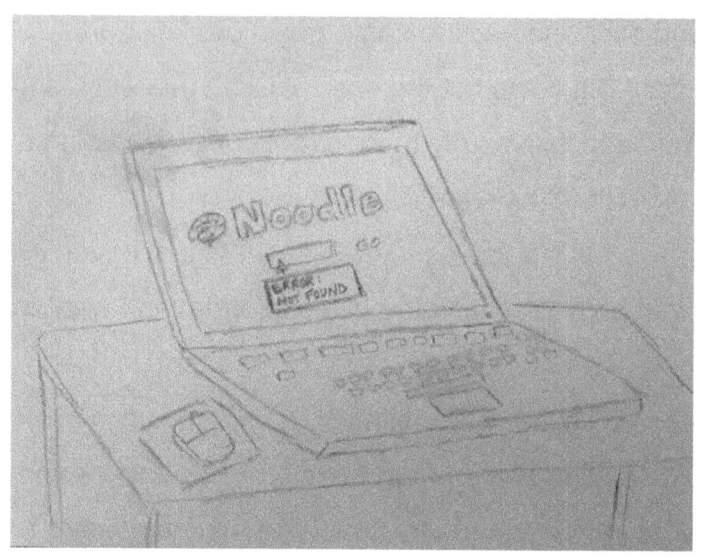

Remember back in the introduction when I talked about what I did for a living prior to the accident? As a reminder, I was a neuroscience nurse practitioner with years of experience taking care of patients with neurological and neurosurgical illness. The irony of this situation was not lost on me at any point in recovery.

6

The fatigue factor

It's amazing how much a human can sleep! For months, I would get my kids up in the morning for school and once they were safely off on the bus, I would go back to sleep for the next 3 hours. It was exhausting getting them all up and out the door. When I would wake up the second time, I would try to do dishes or laundry or something useful and get exhausted and need to lay down for another nap. I figured if I couldn't go to work, I should at least get things done around the house - but I was never able to stay on top of the housework because I was always tired, and any activity wore me out.

I've had insomnia for years that would come and go, but I hadn't had real good sleep since my kids were little. Prior to that point, I was an amazing sleeper - my head would hit the pillow and I'd be out. I've slept through trains shaking my entire house and knocking things off the wall. My parents used to take me to my sisters' band concerts as an infant and I would be sound asleep in my car seat in the front row of the auditorium - that was my sleeping style until I was a parent. That's my partner's sleeping style, still!

After the accident, I was sleeping hard through the night, though not necessarily restful. Well, I was sleeping hard except for the nightmares - I would wake up seeing headlights coming at me. I often had to relive the accident in my dreams, whether I was sleeping during the day or at night. Sometimes it would even happen if I was daydreaming or staring off into space. That made it difficult to get back to sleep - anytime I closed my eyes the headlights were right there again.

I could get all the sleep in the world, and I was still tired. Any activity would wear me out and I'd need a nap. I was falling asleep in the car riding with my family, even on short drives. I was falling asleep on the couch watching TV with the family (I didn't have the TV on much when I was alone, or I probably would have fallen asleep then, too). If I was emotionally or physically stressed, I needed a nap. And when I say emotionally or physically stressed, it did not have to be a life altering event or strenuous workout.

If I had to make a decision of any sort, it was taxing on my brain. Deciding on what to make for dinner, what to eat if we happened to stop at a restaurant or trying to remember something - these were all insignificant things in the grand scheme, but they were hard things to do and would wipe me out. I wasn't able to do actual workouts - PT wanted me to walk a mile most days of the week, and that was quite a feat because of my balance. Going up or down the stairs, doing a load of laundry, washing the dishes - those were all enough to physically wipe me out. I couldn't even consider the big workouts I used to do. I've previously run 13 half marathons and was training for my first full marathon when the accident happened, so I went from regularly working out, to regularly struggling to complete a mile walk.

I'm not much of a coffee drinker because all my life I've been able to fall asleep while drinking coffee, so that wasn't an option to keep me awake now either. In fact, I would make a small pot of coffee just to drink it and forget I even made it (remember the last chapter on memory?).

Ever so slowly, the fatigue started to improve. Eventually, I no longer needed hours of naps, but I still needed rest after activities. At times I could do a quick 30-minute nap and be able to get up and try another activity or finish what I had already started. I was still not able to complete multiple chores at once, however, or go from one activity to another seamlessly. There had to be breaks between activities, or I would 'hit my wall'.

Once the over-sleeping finally calmed down, the insomnia came back due to hyperfocus. I would think and overthink, not being able to stop worrying, overanalyzing, or thinking about all the "what ifs". My mind was constantly going. It would make falling asleep difficult, or I would wake up in the middle of the night and have difficulty falling back to sleep because of it. I would try to listen to music or play a simple mindless game on my phone to distract myself, but nothing worked. In the past, I would have pulled out a book and read until I could get back to sleep, but was still struggling with reading, so that wasn't an option.

I'm not a big fan of sleeping medications because of the side effects and the dependency I've seen in my patients, and I've never been inclined to try them myself because of this. The only thing I would generally recommend to my patients was melatonin, which is a natural hormone in your body that helps you fall asleep and stay asleep. I had previously tried melatonin with no huge improvement, but I was willing to try again. I found a chewable form to try, and it did finally help me get some sleep, though still not perfect sleep.

Six months into recovery, if I attempted bigger activities with more emotional or physical stress, I still required naps up to a couple hours in length. Most of the time I could move forward with a short nap or just some quiet rest time. As I was finally starting to feel a little better, however, I tried pushing the envelope a little - testing my limits, if you will. I tried to see where those new limits were, and when I found them...I needed another 2–3-hour nap. It was frustrating, to say the least.

In a later chapter, I'll talk about our family vacation - it had been booked months before the accident and was largely nonrefundable, so since we all needed a break from real life, we still went. And though I took a lot of breaks and naps on the trip, it still took a week to recover once we were back home. During that week, I struggled with fatigue, more severe headaches, irritability, and more frustration. I was hoping to get back to work after the trip, but it just proved once again that I wasn't ready for regular activities yet.

Sleep started to come up as a point of discussion with all of my therapists. It has been proven that if you get poor sleep or too little sleep during the recovery process, it will slow your recovery. The melatonin was helping a bit, but not a significant amount and the effect decreased over the months that I used it. I'm so sensitive to side effects that I still wasn't up for trying prescription sleep aids. It was time to up the melatonin dose and consider other things that could potentially help me sleep.

Unfortunately, while I knew sleep is essential for brain healing, I had yet to find a trick that would help me sleep. I'm incredibly sensitive to medication side effects, so prescription medications still weren't a viable option for me.

Eight months into recovery, I was still struggling with fatigue, just not to the same extent. If I "hit my wall", I still needed a 2-hour nap to recover, and I seemed to hit it harder than before (as much as I could remember, that is). It didn't happen as often, and I was not requiring naps daily anymore, but my endurance for activities was still very limited and workouts still didn't happen regularly due to this.

In the months to come after this, I did finally find some relief from my insomnia. We upgraded the curtains in the bedroom to blackout curtains and put curtains over the doors outside our bedroom to block out as much light as possible. While historically I could fall fast asleep regardless of the light status or time of day, it appeared now that I needed the room very dark in order to sleep, at least at night. This was the only thing that seemed to make a significant difference in my ability to sleep.

7

The appointment marathon

My phone calendar became my best friend. Since my memory failed me often, I learned to put everything on the calendar. Therefore, if it didn't make it to the calendar, it didn't get done or attended. If I forgot to put something on the calendar, I would find myself the day of or day before the activities getting text messages reminding me of things and I'd have to figure out how to adjust my schedule based on this "new" information.

There were so many activities that I "almost forgot" because I didn't get them on the calendar - they ranged from my therapy appointments to dinner or lunches with friends. I needed time with people but couldn't do much more than the 1-2 hours it would take for lunch or dinner with a friend.

Thankfully they were understanding when I was running late because I "almost forgot" (i.e., I forgot).

Initially getting on the PT and OT schedules were difficult because they were booked, but once we got out a few weeks, PT and OT were weekly events. Both appointments could be held at the same location, so we scheduled them on the same day as much as possible, so I didn't have to drive multiple times. We had to trade off the potential that I could be tired from back-to-back appointments with the fact that I still didn't like driving, even if it was just 20 minutes to the clinic for therapy.

When we were nearing the end of the scheduled appointments and still needed to schedule more, we often couldn't schedule them back-to-back and had to fit them in wherever there were openings, which sometimes meant the appointments required a change in location from my typical office. This is when it became especially difficult to remember which location to go to, even if I had it marked on my phone calendar (which I always did). I found out the hard way that my phone didn't automatically give me reminders for events (I had to set the reminders), but even if it did give me reminders, it just reminded me *of* the event - if I wanted to know the location, I had to click *into* the event to find it.

Seven months into recovery and nearly as long in therapies, I finally had a day where I didn't completely get to the wrong location. I was driving to PT and as usual was heading to my normal clinic, but suddenly I had a thought - 'this was not my normal day I go to PT' (I usually went on Wednesdays and this was a Tuesday), so I had the thought that I just might not be driving to the right location, either. When I had to stop at a stop light, I pulled up the location on my calendar, and sure enough, I was driving to the wrong location.

I called the clinic and explained my dilemma and the scheduler got in touch with my PT - he could still see me at the other location because he had a cancellation after me, so he was still free (it was going to take longer to get to the other location). I took this as a huge win - I remembered *while* I was driving that something was off, rather than getting to the registration desk inside the clinic only to find I was in the wrong place, which had happened entirely too many times.

In addition to my OT and PT appointments, I had my neurology and eye doctor appointments…keeping it all straight was difficult. Trying to read my calendar to see when I could schedule new appointments was also sometimes difficult. I have always prided myself on a color-coded calendar; everything has a specific color. But I couldn't always remember my color-coding, and sometimes I had to take multiple looks at days to make sure they were actually open. Then there were times I would stare at the calendar thinking there was something else that was supposed to be on that day, but I couldn't remember what.

When I needed to add mental health appointments, these appointments were at least virtual so I couldn't mess up the location. We tried to set these on a specific day each week, also, so I wouldn't forget them. I'm thankful that all of the clinics send out reminder texts, too. This way I was less likely to forget them, even if I forgot to put them on my calendar.

8

The journey back to work

Starting right after the accident, it became a bit of a game (though not a fun one), trying to figure out how much time I was going to need off of work. I had a phone call early on with human resources (HR) at work to discuss my options. Do I use my paid time off (PTO) time or go to a short-term disability? How long would I be out? What was going to be the best option? Initially I thought it would just be a day or two off work, so the easy answer was PTO. We would discuss further after I attended some of the appointments and had a better idea what we were dealing with.

When the first couple days passed and I was identifying more issues that would prevent me from going back to work, the answer became a little hazier. I needed to wait to be evaluated by my neurologist, which took a few days to get in. Then I was referred to the eye doctor and PT; I needed to wait to be seen by the eye doctor and get at least the initial PT evaluation done. The eye doctor appointment wouldn't be until the following week, as well as the PT appointment.

Once I was evaluated by the eye doctor, I received the prescription for prism glasses and the referral for OT for vision therapy. Now I needed to order and wait to obtain prisms as well as start the vision therapy before I could get cleared to go back to work. All this while, I still didn't realize how severe everything was - I just wanted to get back to normal life and back to having a regular income.

Once I got the initial appointments with PT and OT completed, we realized how bad my vision and balance really were. I was still incredibly fatigued and headachy and clearly not ready to go back to work, so I needed to wait some more. Days turned into weeks and weeks turned into months.

At some point, the autonomic symptoms became very obvious - they kicked in whenever I was stressed physically or emotionally. Autonomic refers to the nervous system response. When we learned about the autonomic system in physiology during nursing school, we learned about two of the main components - the parasympathetic and the sympathetic systems. The parasympathetic is your 'rest and digest', while sympathetic is 'fight or flight'.

My autonomic system was dysfunctional (often termed 'dysautonomia'), more specifically overactive on the sympathetic side of things. My fight or flight was kicking in with minor triggers, such as the little bit of exercise or brain function I could tolerate. We just didn't realize what it was for quite some time. I didn't know to report these little symptoms, and they didn't seem connected to anything else - I just thought I was tired.

I had a headache that was constantly present. It literally would start as soon as I opened my eyes in the morning and was present until I fell asleep at night. It was severe, and it got worse with any kind of stress. Having had migraines since I was a teenager, you'd think I'd be prepared to deal with headaches, but these were a different beast than my migraines. My migraines had an aura - I would get a warning that they were starting most of the time as I would suddenly become tired and start yawning over and over until the pain started. Then the pain would develop on one side of my head (either right or left in my case, though many people just have it on one side of their head). It would throb, I would get sensitive to lights, sounds, and smells, and it would last a few hours - occasionally it would stretch into the next day. I knew my triggers - lack of sleep or poor sleep, accidental exposure to gluten, or extreme stress, and I could try to avoid these as much as possible to prevent the migraines.

THESE headaches, however, started at the back of my head and eventually engulfed my whole head, would cause pain behind my eyes (especially my right eye), and felt like I had been hit upside the head with a baseball bat. There was no throbbing, no pulsing, just intense pressure. I was always sensitive to lights and sounds now, so that wasn't specific to when the headaches would be at their worst. I couldn't take my migraine medications because these weren't migraines (though I did try once with no effect). Ibuprofen and Excedrin, my typical go-tos, had little effect on the pain, and the one thing I could remember about headache treatment was that I wanted to avoid rebound headaches (also known as medication overuse headaches), so I wasn't about to be taking ibuprofen or Excedrin regularly for the headaches. I reserved these for when the headaches were unbearable, so it would take the edge off.

After months of these headaches and identifying the dysautonomia, my neurologist started me on propranolol, a beta blocker, to hopefully treat the headaches and dysautonomia. He wanted to give this medication a few weeks to work, so we pushed back my start date for work yet again, but hopefully it would do the trick and I would be able to start back at work with a couple of hours a day sooner than later.

Unfortunately, the propranolol was not having its desired effect. I had initial improvement in my headache the first week, but then it just started ramping back up. Within a couple of weeks, I started having swelling (edema) in my legs extending its way up to my knees and I had to stop due to this dangerous side effect. The swelling went down

55

within a few days of stopping, and there was no change in my headache and autonomic symptoms. This was a disappointing experiment.

I was still not tolerating more than a couple of hours of any specific activity, especially if it required brain power. I had gotten approval from my neurologist to start working at 2 hours at a time and gradually increase (pending success with the propranolol noted above), but my work couldn't accommodate bringing me back until I could tolerate 4 hours at a time. Essentially, I'd just be getting into a groove of whatever we were doing at work before the 2-hour limit would hit and it wouldn't be a beneficial use of time. Understandable, but still disappointing.

After 5 months of reporting concerns with my memory since the accident and having the lingering questions of when I could return to work still not answered, I received a referral for neuropsychiatric testing. This would clarify the symptoms that I already knew were there - memory impairments, processing speed issues, and if I wasn't "impaired" according to the testing parameters, I was "borderline", which given my education level and years of experience were "impaired" for me... The neuropsychologist recommended 3 more months off, with additional cognitive therapy (to be done with speech therapy) prior to returning to work. More referrals, which would lead to more appointments, and more time away from work.

As all of the appointments were stacking up, the delays in getting back to work continued, and I continued to work with HR to figure out when I could get back to work and what I needed to do in the meantime to protect my job. I was only there for a month prior to the accident, so I didn't qualify for protection under the family and medical leave act (FMLA).

I used a week of PTO and then went with a short-term disability. As time went by, I used up all 12 weeks of short-term disability. Long term disability was supposed to kick in automatically, but they required a separate review of evidence (even though it was the same company as the short-term disability) and since they didn't receive all the medical records that were requested to show this was not a pre-existing condition, my long-term disability application was automatically denied. I would have to request a formal review to evaluate for a different decision. I didn't understand their letter when it came and had to have Don help me decipher what I needed to do.

I drafted a letter and had Don review it, also, before sending, to make sure it sounded right. I downloaded the last few notes from the neurology clinic, including the neurologist and both PT and OT to include with the letter. The formal review request was sent and fingers crossed. A month went by, and I hadn't gotten any updates. I called a couple of times and finally got a call back noting that all documents had finally been received and the claim would be sent for review. Now I waited again for another response. More time went by, still no responses to more voicemails left. Waiting in limbo without disability checks for 4 months is definitely less than ideal.

I had no legal protection for my job given my lack of qualification for FMLA. That said, my boss kept checking in with me regularly for updates and to tell me the team was looking forward to my return whenever I would be ready, and they would work with me on what that looked like when I get closer to a return date. She reassured me they would keep me on the employment list to increase my chances of getting long term disability coverage.

I was continually amazed at how much my new employer cared about me as a person, especially since I had only been with them for one month. I imagine this would have looked very different had I been with any of the larger institutions I had previously worked for. I am well aware that not everyone has this kind of experience with their employers when an injury occurs.

I started looking into alternate options for finances, since the car insurance payments weren't coming regularly, the disability payments were currently nonexistent, and the bills still needed paying. Our two-income household had dropped to one suddenly, but our bills didn't go down. I looked into unemployment, though I was still technically employed. I learned that I didn't qualify for unemployment in my state because I was not injured at work.

I looked for job postings that may be 'easier' jobs for me to do and reached out to a couple of the listings - they also could not accommodate 2-3 hours at a time, so these weren't options either. In order to pick up anything new, I would have to learn to do something, and as noted in my neuropsychological testing, learning new information was a struggle for me. And so, the financial frustrations continued, and I still didn't have a return-to-work date.

9

Weathering the headache storm

I briefly mentioned the headaches previously. I have a history of migraines dating back to my early teens. This was a family heirloom, it seemed. The first book I published in 2023 was a book to help others reduce their headaches as I had done for myself and countless patients over the years as a nurse practitioner, entitled *Migraine help from a Unicorn Nurse Practitioner*. As noted in my previous book, my migraines largely went away when I cut out gluten years ago. Then they tended only to happen if I slept poorly or if I accidentally ingested gluten.

As stress increased at work prior to my job change, the headaches started being a problem again. In all my years of experiencing migraines, I never had to take preventive medications. I took a lot of vitamins and supplements and managed stress, avoided gluten, and tried to get good sleep. A little over a year prior to the accident, I'm pretty sure I had covid, though I tested negative several times. I was sicker than I've ever been, missed a week of work, and had several months of daily headaches following. Those daily headaches finally went away when I got a daith piercing in my left ear, but this got infected and had to be removed. Luckily, the headaches didn't return as they were prior to the piercing, and I seemed to be back to my baseline with migraines. I do plan to get the daith redone at some point if my migraines ever come back - that was a life saver for me!

After the accident, I experienced eye pressure and eye fatigue that seemed to cause most of my headaches. The headaches literally started as soon as I opened my eyes in the morning and lasted until I went to sleep at night. They varied in intensity throughout the day, but they were always present. Not a day would go by that I didn't have some level of headache present. The headaches would get worse with stress, which would make it even more difficult to think.

If I "overdid" it, the headache would amplify, triggering my autonomic response. I started to use the terms "overdid" or "hit my wall" because clearly, I was doing more than my brain would allow for. It was easy for my family and friends to understand and didn't require any additional explanations. The more I overdid it, or the longer I pushed through whatever activity I was doing, the longer it would take for me to recover.

The headache felt like I was hit upside the head with a baseball bat and the pressure went from the back of my head to the front, with the whole head feeling like it would explode. There was no throbbing like I had with migraines, no unilateral pain, just pain and pressure in the whole head and pain into the eyes (my right eye especially). I presumed the right eye being worse pain was related to the overstimulation to that eye. My typical migraine treatment wasn't working.

After some experimenting trying to find something that would work, energy drinks seemed to be the only thing that would help reduce the headache when it was really bad. I didn't have to take in the entire can, just drink some of it, and only Monster energy drinks worked. I experimented with a few trying to find something with the least amount of sugar and additives, but Monster was the only one that worked for me. I at least got the zero sugar versions, so I didn't have all the sugar calories. And no, I'm not getting paid by Monster, but it sure would be nice if I was!

As I mentioned previously, I tried propranolol, had the initial reduction in headache the first few days, then it ramped up to what it was prior to starting, even as the dose increased. I ultimately had to stop the propranolol because of edema in my legs which cleared up within a few days of stopping the medication again. I felt like I was back to square one.

I felt a little awkward reporting this to my neurologist, but admittedly the only time I would really get relief from the headache was during sex. My neurologist thought this may be related to the parasympathetic system being more responsible for sexual arousal, and supposed it was overcoming the sympathetic response during that time (I'll talk more about the nervous system response in the next chapter). Regardless of the reason, I was sure happy to have one activity that would take away my headache, at least for a little while.

10

Circuit malfunction

As I mentioned previously, dysautonomia or autonomic dysfunction tends to refer to the 'rest and digest' or 'flight or fight' response, in regard to the parasympathetic and sympathetic parts of the autonomic nervous system, respectively. My fight or flight was on overdrive. It would kick in with any kind of physical or emotional stress. I would experience dizziness, increase in the severity of my headache, sweating (sometimes profuse), worsening balance, and slurred speech. When this kicked in, I would require cooling off, physically and emotionally.

I found things that worked by trial and error, because I had no access to my usual knowledge on this subject. I found that drinking ice cold water, eating ice cream, and taking cool showers or using a cold washcloth on my face, neck, and chest (and sometimes my whole body) would help. I also had to get away from stimulation - I had to get to a quiet, dark room, put my noise canceling headphones on, put a hat over head and face to block out the light, and sometimes just went completely under a blanket to block out everything. Later, I found noise canceling earbuds, but when I really 'hit my wall' I sometimes still needed both the earbuds in my ears and the headphones over my ears.

There is a lesser-known portion of the autonomic nervous system, the third pillar, known as the enteric nervous system. This is responsible for gastrointestinal (stomach and bowel) responses to stress. I would later realize that this is what caused my significant stomach upset at times when I significantly hit my wall.

Working with PT, we began following a treadmill protocol during our sessions to gradually increase the treadmill speed and incline every few minutes while monitoring my heart rate and symptoms. We identified that symptoms kicked in when my heart rate got to approximately 110-120, which typically happened somewhere between 13-17 minutes of walking. When that happened, I had to stop and drink cold water and sit down in a chair for symptoms to back off so we could do anything else during my appointment time. The longer the activity, if I tried to push through it, the longer the recovery took.

We used the term 'hit a wall' because it was literally like a switch was flipped and I would go from being fine to not being fine, like I physically hit a wall and could not move forward. The problem was that I didn't realize I had hit the wall until after it was hit. Don got really good at monitoring me, and he reported noticing a change in my whole demeanor - my face went blank, I would stare into space, I would get flushed and start sweating profusely, then the headache would increase, the dizziness came on and the slurred speech. I could typically identify it was happening around the headache time.

The propranolol prescription was supposed to help with this, in addition to the headache I discussed earlier, but it didn't cause any change in my autonomic symptoms prior to having to stop the medication due to the side effects. I did find some relief listening to 8D music. I was introduced to this music prior to the accident as a means to calm down if I was getting anxious (I was experiencing a lot of stress and needed a good outlet).

8D stands for 8 dimensional - think of a 3D movie where it feels like the things on the screen are coming out at you when you put on the special glasses. In the case with 8D music, you put on headphones and listen, or you can lay your cell phone sideways in front of you, to hear the waves of music going from the left speaker to the right and back again. You can find nature music and even more popular songs in this genre of music. Occasionally, I would remember about this new style of music and listen to relax when I was really stressed, and it also helped calm the autonomic effects. Unfortunately, I often forgot about it.

Later on with PT, when autonomic symptoms were brought on during a session, we switched to breathing exercises with calming music and I had a reduction in the headache and palpitations I was experiencing. My PT appreciated when I would remember to wear my smart watch, so we could easily read my heart rate. I happened to have it on when we first introduced the calming music, and we noted reduced heart rate with the calming techniques during the appointment. Technology can be our friends - we just have to remember to use it sometimes!

11

The battlefield within

The longer all of these symptoms and time off work went on, the more my mental health started being affected. My short-term disability paid significantly less than my normal income, so we started having difficulty paying bills and we started digging into our savings (thankfully I had money in my savings account - we had been planning on putting up a fence in the backyard this year for the dogs). Short term disability ended after 12 weeks, then it was supposed to roll into long term disability, per my discussion with HR.

When the short-term disability ended, however, I received a letter that said long term disability had to do their own evaluation to determine eligibility. They needed to determine if my issues were related to a pre-existing condition and needed to obtain medical records to review this. I was a little confused, because this was the exact same company that had just taken care of my short-term disability, so they had my application with the description of why I needed the disability. I had to sign a release of information form for every medical practice and pharmacy I've used for the last 2 years for the company to determine if this was pre-existing or not.

While I continued to go to all of my appointments, I received letters every two weeks to update me that my case was still under review. I received a large packet of information that I had to complete as part of the process, which included yet again having to explain the details of the accident. My PTSD was triggered, and I had autonomic symptoms kick in by the time I finished the packet. After all of this, I received a letter that the claim was automatically denied because they did not receive all of the medical records they requested within the 60-day period.

The letter stated that I could request a formal review, which meant I had to send a letter and any additional documents supporting my case to my case manager. This could be sent by snail mail or by fax, there was no option to send it electronically to expedite the process. I opted for fax to get it there as soon as possible, had to find a place to fax it, and was astonished to pay $24 to fax my letter and the latest notes from PT, OT, and neurology to show I was continuing treatment and it was accident related. After weeks of no response, I called multiple times to try to get an update and had to leave voice messages. When I finally got a call back, I had to answer a couple more questions and be told I had to wait yet again to get an update about the review.

My only other source of income was the car insurance lost wages payout. This did not come weekly like my short-term disability. This required multiple phone calls and documents sent from both my employer and neurologist to show that I was still not back to work. I would call the claim medical representative periodically to check on this and be told they were still waiting on documentation. On two separate occasions, the day after I called for an update (and was told they were still waiting on documentation), I would get a message that I had a payment to accept…but there were so many times that nothing happened, and I continued to wait on payments.

After months of this going on and having my medical claim representative switch on me without notice, I spoke to a supervisor and found out that the clinic bills were not going through the car insurance as they were supposed to be, they went to my primary insurance instead. This meant the car insurance didn't know I was still being treated, even though I was having the clinic send updates directly to them. Apparently at some point I had messed this up by telling the clinic the wrong information at check in.

The insurance supervisor spoke to the billing department at the clinic and all of the visits had to be re-filed through car insurance so they could get all of the related documentation. I was notified by the records department that they were not aware I had been in an accident; they thought all of my appointments were headache follow up. It seemed like a comedy of errors, but it wasn't funny at all. I expressed my concern to my neurologist, and he clarified that his note should easily identify that I was in a car accident and that I had a concussion. He added another treatment code specifically for 'motor vehicle accident' for good measure, even though there were codes already attached to the notes for concussion and diplopia (double vision).

The supervisor from the car insurance told me it's not their responsibility to chase down records for members; it is the responsibility of the member to follow up with clinics to make sure everything was being sent. I explained to her that I had a head injury and couldn't remember everything… her response was, "have you tried writing things down?" Well, this was extremely helpful advice - I hadn't thought of writing anything down until she mentioned this… (cue huge eye roll). I could write down "breathe" on my to-do list and still forget…

I started feeling like a huge burden on my family. My career had me as the primary breadwinner in the home, yet I wasn't able to bring in any significant income. The mortgage and most of the bills were based on my income alone, and my income was nonexistent. In my head, if I couldn't bring in money to support the family, then I should be taking care of things around the house, but I couldn't keep up with chores around the house because of all of my symptoms.

I'm used to constantly moving. I have always been an extremely busy person. Prior to the accident, I worked full time and then some. I had a full-time position and a couple of side gigs going at all times. I had gotten in this mode as a single parent before my significant other and his daughter moved in. Aside from working outside the house, I made dinner most nights and took care of many of the household responsibilities, ran my podcast, and took care of the kids.

The kids did chores every other weekend when they were at our house, but Don and I both have 50/50 custody of our kids, so they're not with us half the time. The kids didn't do much around the house during the week because of school and extracurricular activities. Don had always helped with household activities as he was able around his work schedule (cooking, cleaning, yard work, working on vehicles, etc.) but since the accident he often worked long hours at work, for months was busy with side jobs, and had to get back to taking classes in the fall to complete the degree he was working on, so he wasn't able to help as much as he always had.

I found myself unable to do multiple chores in a row due to fatigue and autonomic symptoms, unable to multitask with essentially anything, and I would forget what I was doing and start another task. If I had to do a lot of stairs as part of the task I was working on (laundry especially since the machines were in the basement), I would burn out faster. Every day I was taking extended naps during the day to recover from whatever I was trying to do.

I started having thoughts that everyone would have been better off had the accident ended differently. If I had died in the accident (which would have been entirely possible), they'd have my life insurance money; it wouldn't matter that I didn't have income. They wouldn't have to worry about if I was doing something or not, and I couldn't screw anything up around the house. In the past, my kids (especially my youngest) didn't have a great relationship with their dad, and I always swore I would never leave them alone without me in their lives. At this time, my kids had a better relationship with their dad, and I felt more confident that he could take care of them just fine without me.

While we had gotten engaged prior to the accident happening, I started to feel like Don *had* to stay with me and didn't have a choice. He had told me that he felt like it was his fault that I was injured because he was the driver in the accident. He joked that "he broke me, so he bought me", like the saying if you break something at the store. I didn't see it as a joke regardless of how many times he insisted it was, so I felt like he couldn't leave me after the accident since I was broken. I didn't feel like he was staying with me because he *wanted* to, but rather because he *had* to - he had an obligation to me since 'he broke me'. He always said this wasn't true, but my brain was telling me otherwise.

My 'fuse' was much shorter than it had ever been. My humor didn't seem to be the same. Things I would have laughed at and joked about before no longer seemed funny. Don and I always used to be able to joke about things, which was one of the favorite things we both had about our relationship. Things we would have argued with previous partners about were literally just jokes to us. We didn't get mad at these little things - we could laugh at them and see them for the minutiae that they were. This seemed to be gone. I started getting upset and taking these jokes personally, which only caused tension between Don and me. It was like I forgot how to laugh.

In general, I didn't feel like the same person I was prior to the accident. Not even a little bit. There was nothing that I do now that was as easy or as well done as it used to be prior to the accident. Yes, I could still cook, but I burned things a lot or ruined the food because I forgot about it on the stove or in the oven. I missed steps in recipes even though I read them multiple times, never mind the fact that I had to even use recipes for things I've made many times.

Yes, I could still do laundry, but I forgot to change it over much more often than ever before and would have to rewash clothes because they got musty in the washer. I forget to look for things in pockets like chapstick or pens and would have clothes come out stained or ruined because of it. I didn't separate clothes out correctly and accidently put things in the dryer that were supposed to be laid flat to dry or things that I previously wouldn't have put in the dryer just for the fact that they lose their soft texture.

I have run 13 half marathons and was supposed to run my first full marathon a couple of months after the time of the accident. I was running multiple times weekly and doing strength training on other days during the week, typically taking 1-2 days off of exercise each week. Initially after the accident I couldn't walk more than a mile before autonomic symptoms stopped me. It took six months to get up to 3-3.5 miles at a time (not every day) but only on flat surfaces - if there were hills, I was still done sooner.

I couldn't get through a full 30-minute workout without having to take breaks and modify all the moves due to balance and fatigue and autonomic symptoms. My exercise routine has been a constant in my life for over a decade, and I prided myself in all that I could do. That seemed like distant history now. When I would focus on getting my walks or limited exercise in daily, I would forget to do the exercises from PT and OT, and when I focused on getting my exercises done for PT and OT, I would forget to get my walks or limited exercise in.

Yes, I could still clean, but I couldn't see the details and could only do one project at a time. If I did the dishes, I had to rest before I could wipe down the countertops and clean the stovetop and would sometimes have to re-wash dishes because I didn't get them clean the first time. I couldn't multitask and have laundry going at the same time, because if I stopped to change over the laundry, I needed to rest before I could get back to what I was doing...and by that time I often forgot what I was doing. The to-do list seemed never ending and while I loved my checklists, the lists never got completed from one day to the next. Things were always spilling over to the next day, and I'd have to triage what really needed to get done the next day because there were inevitably things already on tomorrow's list. So, I stopped using lists because they caused more anxiety than they were helpful.

I used to be able to drive wherever I wanted, whenever I wanted. I've taken my kids on week-long camping trips where we drove from one state park to another all week or halfway across the country to go to a national park, and I've been the only licensed driver in the car. Initially after the accident I could drive 30-60 minutes before my headache significantly increased. I've increased my driving time from a max of 1 hour to a max of 1.5 hours before my headache becomes too much from focusing on the road and everyone around me.

This did not increase my independence very much, as I still couldn't go for longer drives, and needed someone to go with me when my youngest had to be dropped off at summer camp at the end of summer, months after the accident.

I couldn't multitask at all; if someone would speak to me while I was trying to focus on something, I would lose my train of thought on what I was doing and still couldn't recall what the person said to me. If multiple conversations were happening at once, it made focusing on any of them near impossible. We were with friends one night playing cards and multiple conversations were happening in the room as we all sat at a long table. I couldn't track any of the conversations, nor the directions I was getting from the person sitting next to me on how to play the card game (which, by the way, was a game I had played before).

I couldn't read a book - it took a lot of work to visually focus on what I was reading - the lines often didn't even look straight, but also, I had to read the same information over and over to remember what I just read, and I had trouble comprehending what I read. This made reading recipes difficult and remembering the order to do things or following directions to put something together.

We borrowed a carpet shampooer from a friend, and I tried to follow the directions on how to assemble the carpet shampooer. I read the bullet points over and over and still couldn't figure out how to put the dang thing together. This left me as a puddle on the floor crying. I could not comprehend the steps even after reading them multiple times, and still didn't get it put together correctly, so that when we lifted it up to go up the stairs it fell apart. I then couldn't figure out how to actually use the shampooer, and finally Don had to take over.

I felt completely incompetent. I have been a provider taking care of patients for years, diagnosing and explaining complicated neurological conditions, yet here I was unable to figure out how to put together a carpet shampooer and clean my carpet.

As a neurological provider, I used to recommend to my patients if they were struggling with reading after a head injury that they listen to an audiobook instead. I found, however, that while I couldn't focus to read a book, I also couldn't follow to listen to an audiobook. I couldn't focus on the words or the meaning of the words they were using - it seemed to go too quickly but slowing down the speed didn't help either. I couldn't remember what I just listened to, and certainly couldn't do anything else while I was trying to listen. I used to listen to audiobooks and podcasts in the car on my way to and from work. There was no way I could now focus on driving AND focus on whatever I was trying to listen to.

Medical knowledge seemingly slipped my mind. I couldn't remember the names of medications, doses of medications, or anatomy that I've known for 24 years. Some things were still there, but so much just seemed to be gone. Even when I've been out of work for 3 months following foot surgery years ago and post c-section with my last baby, I never lost the knowledge. Sure, I was a little rusty with the charting when I got back to work, but I never lost the knowledge of how to diagnose and treat patients.

Periodically throughout the years I've had friends and relatives reach out with medical questions. I could always answer their questions and give recommendations. Now I was finding myself apologizing and telling them I couldn't remember, and I didn't have access to my work resources to look things up. That said, I doubt I would have been able to look anything up because I just couldn't comprehend the information. I worked so hard to become a nurse practitioner, and I did not at all feel like a nurse practitioner anymore. I was quickly starting to think I would never be a nurse practitioner again, but I would still have to finish paying off my school loans.

I couldn't tolerate busy places. With all of the noise, lights, people moving everywhere and multiple conversations happening, I would get overwhelmed and hit my wall. I got tunnel vision and couldn't focus on anything when there was too much noise, and then the noise just seemed louder. I started wearing my noise canceling headphones to my children's events, and this seemed to help a bit.

My middle child is in a swim club and the indoor swim meets were extremely loud. I learned to stay out of the pool area except for when he was actually swimming, and if I went in with my headphones on, I could watch his race and leave again to try to survive the whole swim meet. We would camp out in another area of the facility, and I brought our camp chairs with us - there were multiple times I took a nap between races. If I pushed past my wall, however, not even the noise canceling headphones would block out the sound anymore. Later on, I found noise canceling earbuds, so they weren't as obvious, but they worked the same as the headphones for blocking sound, and when I was really bad, I needed to use both at the same time.

I've had a loss of my peripheral vision. I used to have extremely good peripheral vision, despite my historically poor eyesight. Since the accident, however, I couldn't see everything in my periphery. My field of view narrowed, and I noticed what seemed like blind spots. When doing the computer testing with OT, I would completely lose sight of the arrows on the screen and have to move my head around to find them again.

When I noticed this, my first thought was that I had a visual field cut (literally meaning loss of areas of my visual field) like I used to see with my stroke patients, and it was very alarming. My OT explained that it was likely happening because my brain was stressed and compensating by narrowing my field of vision, and that the exercises we were doing would hopefully desensitize the brain to all the overstimulation so these blind spots would decrease. While driving, I have missed entire vehicles in my periphery, and it startles me when I finally see them. I would also forget to look in my blind spots, which certainly didn't help me to overcome these decreased visual fields.

I've had a loss of my regular vision, not just the periphery. As I mentioned earlier, I've had bad eyesight all of my life, but I have done so much better since my surgeries 10 years ago. With my vision knocked off course, my current prescription glasses were not helping. The new trouble with double vision required me to get prism glasses. The prisms initially helped to clear up vision for driving but seemingly nothing else.

After going through all the changes with the eye patch and tape and the dot on my glasses, my right eye started working like it did before I had LASIK done after my lens implants. If I closed my left eye, nothing seemed clear, and everything seemed darker. My degree of double vision meant it was not clearly two overlapping objects, but it was not singular objects, either. This made everything difficult - including trying to read words, letters, or numbers across a line when working with OT, holding steady to write my signature or to try making an entry in my journal, and staying within the lines when coloring.

In the fall of 2022, months before the accident, I started my own podcast as part of my Brain Wellness business, sharing my knowledge on neurological conditions with anyone who would listen. Prior to changing jobs, I recorded plenty of interviews to get me through to the fall - literally months of interviews were already on my computer. I was thankful for this when I started the new job because it meant I could focus on my orientation and just release the interviews weekly rather than having to spend time recording them after a long day of work.

Following the accident, there was no way I could have recorded a podcast. When I would get stressed or tired, I would start slurring my words and my word finding difficulty was exaggerated. When I tried to talk a lot, I started struggling with word finding even more and didn't feel intelligent because of it. Sometimes I couldn't come up with simple words, but I could try to explain the word I was looking for and make a lot of hand gestures to try to help whomever I was talking to understand what I was trying to say.

Even though all I had to do each week was post a teaser clip and post the announcement for the episode, this still was more work than anticipated. It took longer to process anything related to the podcast, including finding a 20-30-second clip to use as a teaser, remembering to post the teaser and the announcement, even remembering where they were saved on my computer week after week even though it was the same activity. I was still getting emails from people I had lined up for interviews, which were now postponed until I felt ready, and I had difficulty remembering to respond to these emails.

As part of my Brain Wellness business, I also would go live on social media once a week to share a brief wellness topic, which I called Wellness Wednesday. I haven't recorded a Wellness Wednesday since the accident for the same reasons as noted above. I didn't even reach out to friends or family to talk on the phone because I didn't feel intelligent when I spoke. I hated how much I struggled to come up with words, and I hated when I would stutter trying to find the next part of my sentence or thought. The more anxious I became, the worse it got.

This all was starting to compound, and I started having very dark thoughts. I started having more thoughts of wishing the accident had ended differently. I felt more and more of a burden and felt completely incompetent at life. I didn't just have difficulty multitasking, I had difficulty just tasking.

One day, I had an episode where I was feeling panicky and for once actually recognized it as a panic attack. I thought about taking one of my anti-anxiety medications, but for a split-second thought that maybe I should just take the whole bottle and be done with this whole experience, be done being a burden. Then I was scared that I had the thought and scared of even opening the bottle, so I didn't take any of my medication and just battled through the panic attack, crying myself to sleep. I didn't tell anyone about this episode and hoped it would just go away.

Then I had another episode where I was overwhelmed with everything, on edge, and I went to my room to lay down. I put the pillow over my head to block out all the noises and lights and for a split second realized I was holding the pillow too tight because I couldn't breathe. Then for another split second I had a thought that it wouldn't be such a bad thing if I just held the pressure like that until all the sounds and lights went away completely. Then I was scared that my mind went there again and feared just how easy it would have been to continue with the action.

This made me cry even harder. Eventually Don came into the room and found me sobbing and came to me, asked me what was wrong, and I told him what had happened through my ragged sobbing. He just held me and prayed for me until I stopped sobbing and ultimately fell asleep in his arms.

At that point I realized I needed help, and I couldn't get myself out of this situation. I had had times of what I called 'situational depression' in the past, revolving around divorce and moves and major transitions in life. A previous therapist had called this 'adjustment disorder' instead of 'situational depression' because it wasn't truly depression. In these previous disordered episodes, I had never had dark thoughts like this, and the feelings were always self-limiting. It would take me a few months and the feelings of sadness would resolve. This new mental health state was something I had never experienced, and it was scaring the crap out of me.

Sometimes brain injuries cause debilitating symptoms that cause the person to feel depressed. After a stroke, for example, if someone loses their ability to move one side of their body or speak, this can cause depression because they can't function like they used to. It's a completely understandable response to the situation. Sometimes brain injuries cause depression just because the chemistry of the brain is altered from the injury - no physical symptoms must even be present for this to happen. This response almost seems unreasonable to people who are not experiencing the brain injury - it doesn't make sense why it would be there...but it's just as real as the physical symptom related type of depression.

I knew a general psychologist was not going to have the background needed with the specific troubles I was having (believe me, I tried one and it didn't go well because she had *no* idea what I was going through), so I looked up mental health providers experienced with TBI and sent a couple of messages off to the providers I found near me. A couple days later I had still received no return messages, so I finally tried calling the providers' offices instead only to find out they weren't taking new patients. One of them called me back and gave me referrals for a couple of other practitioners I could reach out to. One of the referred clinics had a therapist that just happened to have an appointment the next day because of a cancellation, so I took it. I didn't want to wait any longer. I *couldn't* wait any longer.

I started working with her about three months into my recovery. I nearly maxed out the scores on both the depression and anxiety screenings at my first appointment with her - these are not scores you want to aim high on. She first verified with me that I had no suicidal plans and helped me identify that what I was experiencing with my scary thoughts were known as "intrusive thoughts". I was still meeting with her weekly, several months later, and we re-evaluated these scores every couple of weeks.

One of the main issues she identified was PTSD. She didn't believe I truly have depression, but instead PTSD from the accident was causing depressive feelings, anxiety, and had heightened my OCD. I started worrying about things constantly, thinking and overthinking about the worst-case scenarios - I would create things in my head to worry about, essentially. I would get overwhelmed when I started to think about all the things I needed to do and become paralyzed, unable to do anything.

Everything made me anxious, and I became hypervigilant - if Don didn't get home exactly when I thought he would, I started to worry that something happened or that he was avoiding me because of how negative I had become and how much stress I was causing on him. My mind would start obsessing over things that weren't actually *things*, at all.

My therapist is certified in art therapy. When we began working together, she wanted me to draw and/or paint what various emotions looked like to me, since all I was experiencing was fear. I used to draw and paint a lot so this seemed like something I could do. I went to the craft store and bought painting supplies. I couldn't wrap my head around the assignment, however, and never got started. I have never done well with abstract thinking. She wanted me to portray the emotions with colors and images that I associated with each emotion. This was something my brain just could not do. The supplies are still sitting in a pile in the corner of my dining room because I still can't comprehend what to do with them.

The next assignment she wanted me to try was to portray what life used to look like versus what life looked like now. She suggested I just try to draw it, since I struggled with the previous assignment. So, I again went to the craft store and this time brought home a sketch book and a pack of pencils. It took me a few days, but I finally got some inspiration and drew a split image with me as a provider and me in a bed in the dark. When I completed the image, I was amazed at how I had captured my feelings so well.

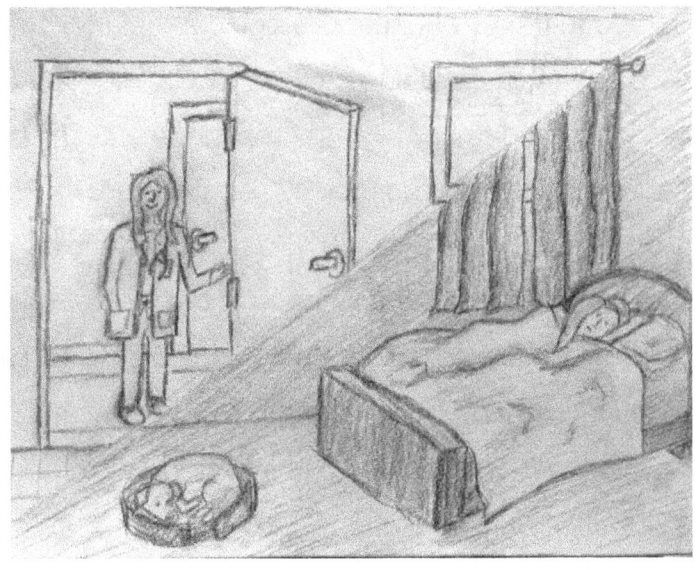

It made me proud that I was finally able to come up with something. I took a picture of my drawing and sent it to a few of my close friends who were aware of my struggles (I had finally opened up to a few people when I realized I couldn't do this on my own anymore) and showed the image to my immediate family. It made a few of them emotional to see what was inside my head. I don't think anyone realized how much I was struggling emotionally until they saw this drawing.

My therapist continued giving me assignments each week. I started keeping them in a note page on my phone, but I would forget they were on my phone and ultimately would forget that I was supposed to be working on assignments. I started writing them on a piece of paper near my spot on the couch so they would be more visible - that helped for a while until I misplaced the notebook I was keeping them in. Sometimes I would find the notes and try to work on the assignments again, often paralyzed by my inability to come up with imagery to describe my feelings.

My therapist still wanted me to try to get the feelings assignment done that she had initially given me and would occasionally ask me about it. She wanted me originally to take one feeling at a time and create an image using colors that I would associate with that feeling and images that I would associate with it. I still struggled with that, as I couldn't think abstractly. However, after a few more days, I finally had thoughts come to mind that conveyed more of my emotions.

The first was my feeling of isolation, of being left out. The best thing I could come up with was my feeling of being left out of the cool surgical cases that I should have been in the week after my accident. I was scheduled to be in the OR for more observation days (the one the day of the accident wasn't initially on my schedule, but since I was shadowing the surgeon who was doing the surgery, I got to join him). As my vision refused to improve and I continued missing more time from work, I started feeling like I might never get back into the OR. And to be honest, I still feel a bit like this, as I have no guarantee that my visual difficulties will correct themselves.

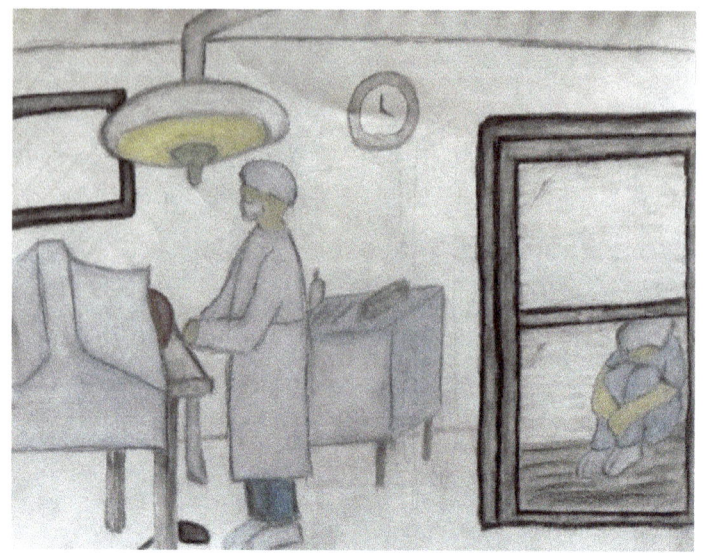

The next emotion I was able to draw was my feeling of being useless. Though my family and friends kept telling me I was not, in fact, useless, I still felt like I was. I couldn't bring in money to support the family and I couldn't get the housework done, so what good was I? I was about as useful as someone painting a house that was on fire - it was an exercise in futility.

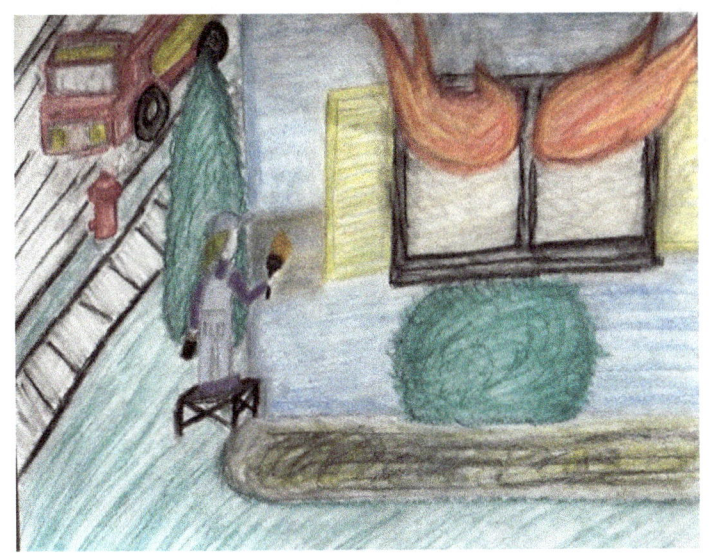

I couldn't shake this feeling, and to some extent still struggle with it as I still have to modify everything I do and can't offer help to others as I'd like. My parents are getting up there in age and need help around their house - I have time to help them but I don't have the stamina to drive to their house, help lift or move a bunch of things, and then drive back home. So, I help with small amounts only, rarely, though I know they need more than I can offer.

For a long time after this last drawing, I couldn't create anything new. I would open my sketch pad and try to turn my thoughts into images but couldn't get it right. I have two incomplete drawings in my sketch book because I just couldn't connect the thoughts. I struggled with them for a long time before I finally just gave up and set the sketch book aside.

One of the biggest assignments my therapist gave me that I could remember was to look for the positives. I was so easily focusing on the negatives in my life, but the positive things were harder to see. Yes, there were positives. I was able to attend my middle child's middle school graduation. I was able to attend my youngest child's talent show on the last day of school. I was able to spend time with my kids over the summer, even if I didn't feel like it was truly quality time. The negatives just out shadowed anything positive I could find.

Nearly every night, we would all sit at the table as a family for dinner, and we would start the dinner by saying what our favorite part of the day was. I had started this tradition years prior when my family was struggling, and we enjoyed the activity. I began hating when it was my turn to say my favorite part of the day, and I loved when I was skipped or forgotten, because I struggled so much coming up with a positive thing to say.

I found myself avoiding getting together with people. I wouldn't reach out to friends or family because I felt that all I did was talk about the negative things in my life. Then I felt like my friends were avoiding reaching out to me because of my negativity. Whether this was true or not, my brain thought it was. All of my friends' and family members' lives kept moving forward - they were changing jobs, getting promoted, or just working their regular hours, while I was just here at home not able to participate in life. I got frustrated when people would tell me they were unhappy at their jobs and didn't want to go. I started to seriously miss adult interaction and wished daily that I *could* go to work and do normal things.

I was home with my kids all summer long, but I didn't feel like I was present. I always had a headache, so I needed them to be quiet. I couldn't tolerate very long walks with them because there was always so much conversation happening - the boys tend to talk about Pokémon the entire walk

105

(the littlest especially). I couldn't exactly ask them not to talk on the walks, though, because that was completely boring for them and then they wouldn't want to go at all.

I often had to send them off to play outside or in another area of the house instead or have them quietly playing electronics (ultimately too much time spent on this) near me so that I could have a quieter environment. At times I would take them to a park or beach or something, but we could only be there for short amounts of time because I would get overstimulated and need to leave.

I missed my friends, but I also didn't want to be around people. It was overwhelming trying to do life with others around, but I was also getting so lonely. I missed out on an opportunity to help a friend, and this troubled me. I had a friend who was struggling with her life. She had been diagnosed with breast cancer and was going through treatment. I watched her social media posts, and they were gut wrenching. She wanted interaction with people as she was going through chemo and had her double mastectomy; she was lonely and wanted to get together with people, but she requested no negativity because she was struggling with her own thoughts. I didn't feel like I could get together with her because all I could do was focus on the negativity in my life and what I couldn't do, and I struggled to see the positive in life.

I thought she was better off without my company than having me there talking about what I couldn't do anymore. She committed suicide and I took it hard. I felt somewhat responsible because I didn't reach out to her when I knew she needed help. I felt guilty for not keeping her company when I clearly had time to do so, and I was scared because my thoughts had led me to a similar dark place, and I didn't really want to go there. I kept retreating further and further inside myself.

I didn't realize how much I identified with my nurse practitioner (NP) role. I used to think it was just part of who I was, but now that I haven't been able to do it, I feel like I've lost it. I started realizing I was feeling grief over the loss of my identity as a NP, even though it hasn't been taken away from me completely yet.

My therapist and a few of my friends started asking me what I would do if I can't get back to my same position. And I honestly don't know what else I will do if I can't get back to it. Healthcare is all I've done since I was 20 years old in 1999, and I have been in neurosciences since 2000 in some capacity. I put so much work into becoming a NP and created so much debt from all of my schooling. I still have to pay off all that debt even if I can't get back to being a NP, and that thought is disheartening, too.

When I finally opened up to Don about all of my emotions, his needs helped pull me out of my dark thoughts. When I explained to Don why I felt like a burden, why I felt like he and the kids were better off without me, he corrected me. Had I died in the accident, not only would he not have me anymore (the most important piece he says), but he would have lost the car and wouldn't have been able to get a new one because his credit score was not as good as mine. His name is not on the mortgage, so he would have lost the house we live in and wouldn't have been able to afford to keep it on his income alone even if he would have been on the mortgage.

Don would have lost out on life with my boys because they would have gone back to their dad permanently. His daughter had moved in with us full time during the summer after the accident, and she was only going to be able to attend school here if she lived in the school district, so if they had to move, she would lose her school and he likely would not be able to keep her with him full time. The rest of this story will come later, but we ended up getting married during my recovery. So, after we got married, he would have taken on the responsibility for my school loans, as well. All of this would financially ruin him, not to mention break his heart.

Then, we talked about how it would affect my kids if I weren't here anymore. I have been the preferred parent for my youngest, especially, since he was born, so losing me would devastate him. My youngest has autism and he likes his structure; he likes the security he feels with me. I don't really want to think about how losing me would have affected him. Yes, the boys' relationship was better with their dad than it was previously, but they still need their mom, too. Deep down, I knew this, but it was hard to rationalize to my damaged brain when I was at my lowest of lows. I finally decided I needed to figure out a way to make life work because ending it would not be an option.

12

Struggling aftermath

Post-traumatic stress disorder (PTSD) showed up right away the day we bought our replacement vehicle. I mean, honestly it showed up a little when I had to get back into a car to go home from the ER, but it really showed up on day 2 after the accident when we drove our new vehicle home from the dealership. When I drove home from the dealership, I should say, and I wasn't even driving the new vehicle - I was driving my vehicle that I've had for several years; Don took the new vehicle that day.

Just the act of driving *any* vehicle put me into a tailspin. This didn't make sense to me - I was the passenger in the accident, not the driver. I would have thought I would struggle more being the passenger again, but I felt safer with Don behind the wheel than by myself.

Initially it was any time in the car, no matter where I went. If there was any intersection involved, my heart was racing. More specifically, anytime I would drive through the intersection where we got in the accident, I would start having a panic attack. I would cry every time I had to drive through said intersection. If I had to stop for a red light there, the crying got more severe, and the anxiety was bigger.

Over time, this very slowly improved to just my heart racing and minimal tears (unless, of course, I had to stop for a red light). It was months before we could try to go to that restaurant again (even though we never made it to the restaurant on the night of the accident), and when we did finally go, I was crying so hard after going through the intersection that I had to wait to calm myself down in order to go into the restaurant when we got there.

Anytime I would see another accident on the road, I had flashbacks from our accident and started crying, regardless of the severity or the location of the accident. Even if I saw someone pulled over, my heart raced at the sight of an emergency vehicle. If an ambulance went by me with lights and sirens on, my heart started racing and I started seeing images from our accident. Even if there were no lights and sirens, just seeing the emergency vehicle next to me set off palpitations.

As innocent as it was, Don was trying out a new video game one day. He was driving a car, racing around corners. His car went around a corner and another car came out of nowhere and ran into him. The headlights, the sound of crashing...I had to leave the living room and go into our bedroom crying. If I was watching any TV show or movie with the family and someone got in a car accident, I would lose it. It would trigger flashbacks and I would have no control over my emotions. I would wake up in the middle of the night with flashbacks from the accident and I would see headlights coming at me. It was not easy to get back to sleep after that happened.

A few months following the accident and purchase of our new Highlander, we realized my PTSD seemed to be at its worst when riding in the new Highlander. Even though we got the same vehicle because of the safety features, I felt the least safe in this vehicle compared to our other small SUV. Honestly, just seeing another of these vehicles on the road made my heart race - especially if it was the same color as ours. More and more I was avoiding our Highlander and opting for our other vehicle, but this was our family vehicle and was the most comfortable for all the kids. Ultimately, we had to make a trip back to the car dealership to trade the Highlander off for something else. I just couldn't stay in it.

We talked about what kind of vehicle we wanted to get, and we had always said our next purchase would be a truck. Don had trucks in the past and we definitely wanted something that could haul our trailer and someday the boat we always dreamed about. So, there was no better time than the present to get the truck. We found a good used one that came out to about the same price as our Highlander so our debt ideally would not increase by much. Unfortunately, interest rates had gone up, but the tradeoff of me being more comfortable in the vehicle for a slightly higher monthly payment was worth it to Don, so we made the trade.

The truck turned out to be the place I felt safest on the road. I sat up higher, it had more muscle than our smaller SUV, I felt like I was more visible to other cars. Maybe it was just a mind trick, but I was going to take any win I could.

At the start of this book writing experience, I was five months into recovery, and I could drive through the intersection without a massive panic attack, but I would still cry. The longer I had to spend at the intersection the harder I would cry, and if I saw another accident anywhere, it was still a struggle. I was on the interstate one day when traffic suddenly came to a stop. Emergency vehicles started coming up the road with sirens on. I tried to steady myself, but I couldn't control it - I started crying. There was no exit close by for me to get off the road and take another route.

I was stuck in the line of cars that was headed directly toward where the emergency vehicles were going. By the time I got up to the accident and saw the crunched cars (there were cars displaced on both sides of the interstate), I was hyperventilating and sobbing. As I was stopped in traffic, I tried sending a couple of text messages to find someone I could talk to, but no one was responding. I was able to stop crying by the time I got home but my autonomic symptoms had kicked in and I couldn't stop sweating. I took a cool shower to try to cool off and still was sweating for about 20 minutes after I got out. In my head, I was right back at the scene of our accident, and I was in panic mode.

I started having what felt like separation anxiety. I didn't like being in groups of people, but I also didn't like being alone. I worried when Don didn't get home when he said he was going to be home. I knew traffic could be awful, and sometimes he would stop at the grocery store or the hardware store on his way home (he may or may not tell me about these stops prior to stopping), and while these were all completely innocent reasons to not be home at the moment I thought he should be, my head was all over the place. I started to worry whether something happened to him at work, or in traffic, or wondered what else could be holding him up from getting home. I would think and I overthink, and I obsessed about all possible horrible outcomes until I would see him pull into the driveway.

I also started having social anxiety. I used to be a social butterfly - I loved getting out of the house, getting together with friends either for bonfires and games at their homes or out to a bar with live music or karaoke. Since the accident, I strongly disliked these activities. My middle child had a picnic for his swim club over the summer - once we got there I so badly wanted to leave. I set up our chairs away from other people and I hoped to avoid conversation with anyone while we were there.

Going to restaurants with my family didn't sound like fun to me, much less going to a restaurant with a group of people. My family has a gathering in the fall every year - we went but I stayed outside most of the day. I felt bad not sitting inside and conversing with everyone, but there's no way we could have stayed as long as we did so my kids could enjoy time with their cousins had I stayed inside.

When it came time for the holidays, I made the hard decision to not take my husband and kids to my family's Thanksgiving celebration. We instead stayed at home and did Thanksgiving with our little family - all the kids and Don helped make the meal and we enjoyed relaxing together and playing games. It was a very peaceful holiday, though I did feel bad we weren't with the extended family.

We did go to my sister's house for our Christmas celebration, however, 8 months post-accident. I was grateful I had brought my noise canceling earbuds, and I had to sneak away to a comfy chair for a nap while we were there. I still didn't get to converse with everyone as I usually would, and I definitely hit my wall by the time we left. I had to take another nap on the drive home, and the headache and irritability spilled into the next day.

My anxiety in general has gone through the roof. I used to have times when I would overthink things, but it turned into a daily occurrence. If there was a thought to be had, there was a thought to overthink to death. I worried about everything, all the time, and had difficulty rationalizing things. I would pace and fidget - things I never used to do. Don called me out on how I was unable to sit still; my leg was always bouncing when we were sitting on the couch together, or at the dinner table with the family, or riding in the car. You would think I would lose some weight with all the pacing and fidgeting I did, but that wasn't happening, unfortunately.

Disability is a lonely place. I wanted to be with people, but I didn't, all at the same time. I didn't want others to see my inability to come up with words or wonder why I couldn't keep up with the conversation. And whether I shared my symptoms and feelings with friends or family or not, I never really felt like they understood what I was experiencing. All summer I had the kids home with me, but I didn't feel present with them.

I craved meaningful interaction with others, but I couldn't grasp it. Only after I started feeling better could I put into words what this felt like. I couldn't come up with a drawing that would do it justice, but I took a stab at poetry - something else I used to write a lot in my younger years. This is what

119

I came up with to express the loneliness of trying to recover from a brain injury:

All alone with the kids on the couch
All alone with my friends at the bar
All alone sitting next to my husband
All alone as I cry in the car

All alone in a room full of people
All alone as I'm lying in bed
All alone though I'm not really alone
All alone with the thoughts in my head

All alone with my injured brain
All alone while I wait to heal
All alone as I lose who I am
All alone is all that I feel

I started to get easily angered. I guess I can't say I've ever been a super calm person. I suppose I've always had a bit of a temper, but it was never anything like it was starting to be. I would get irritated with everything - the kids, the dogs, traffic, people in the store, people on social media, radio personalities, Don, and the list went on. Things I used to find funny weren't funny anymore. When the kids or Don did something silly, I used to laugh about it with them and we would pick on each other (completely in jest, no ill feelings about the things we were saying), but now these things weren't funny, they were annoying, and I had no time for them.

I had no patience, and I had no fuse. I started blowing up over things I generally would not get upset about, and it took me much longer than it should to cool back down. This led to picking fights with Don, something we also generally have not done (we had two, maybe three arguments in two years prior to the accident), then I would get angry with myself for fighting about stupid things. It was a vicious cycle.

In addition to being angry, I became fearful of everything. I became afraid of how long it was taking me to heal. I started to worry that maybe I'll never get back to where I was before. Having been a neurology NP as long as I have, I've seen people recover at various rates. I've seen people get better in a matter of days, weeks, months, years, and I've seen people not get better after their head injuries and they are left with permanent deficits.

The longer it went on, the more I worried I would be one of those people that never gets back to normal. I was also afraid of going back to work and failing. I was only at my new job for one month and my colleagues barely got to know me and what I had to offer the team. Now I didn't have the memory I used to and couldn't seem to access my medical knowledge. I didn't feel qualified to go back to my job, and don't know that I ever will, despite everyone telling me they believe I will.

The one thing I had going for me in all of this was that I changed jobs to a place where I felt like I was family on day one. I felt like I had known these people forever, and they were my people. My boss still checks in with me regularly to see where I am in my recovery, not because she is trying to rush me back, but because she genuinely cares. The team wants me to be able to come back in whatever capacity I can, whenever I'm able.

I was hired as a hospital rounder, which meant I would be covering all of our patients that were in the hospital, following them after surgery as well as evaluating new patients that we were asked to see. I was hired to work at our level 1 trauma hospital, and we were getting ready to take over all of the trauma calls shortly after I started. This job was going to be a demanding one, and I was excited for the challenge…before the accident.

After the accident, with all the sensitivities I've developed to lights and sounds and too much commotion, the idea of rounding in a busy hospital seems outright scary. My boss offered that I could come back in a clinic position instead of the hospital, at least to start, as the pace is slower, and it may help me acclimate better. She also offered that if I don't feel ready for a provider role right away, they might be able to bring me back at first into a nurse role if I need less responsibilities. While it's great to know they are willing to be so accommodating, I worry about going back to either of these roles and not succeeding and feeling like even more of a failure if I can't do these less-intense positions. I have felt like I'm failing at everything and can't stop the spiral very well.

Again, only after I started feeling better was I able to start putting some of these thoughts into images that symbolized how I felt. This one was profound. I spent 6 months trying to gain access to any part of my brain that could be useful, but I felt like my brain was locked up and I was searching through a huge ring of keys trying to find the right one to open the lock.

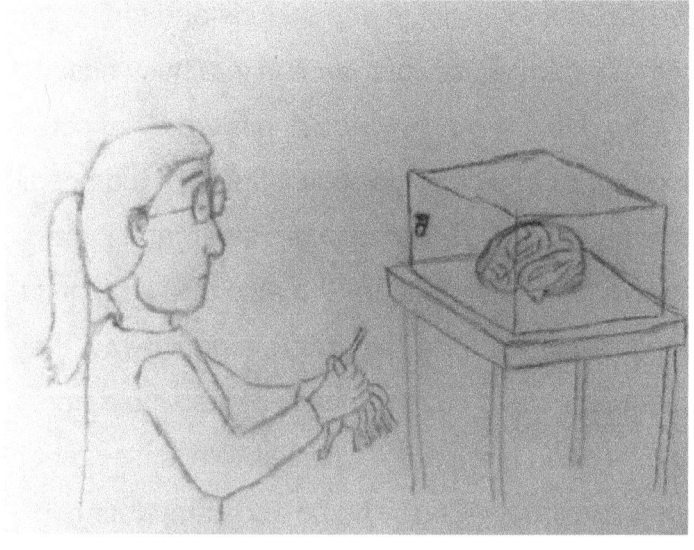

Working in neurology for as long as I have, I'm aware that depression can cause memory issues, but I'm also aware that people with memory difficulties tend to have some level of depression because of it. The two concepts are often intertwined, but at some point, it's like the chicken and the egg - you must try to figure out which of the two is more responsible.

I finally asked my mental health provider if she thought my depression was causing my memory to not improve or if she thought my memory not improving was causing my depression - she thought at that point that it was likely my symptoms not improving that was preventing my mood from improving. So, the next step was getting neuropsychological testing completed, which identified fairly significant impairments in memory and processing, likely the cause of my depression.

13

The voyage to 'I do'

A week before the accident, Don had gotten down on one knee and asked me to be his wife. After a shocked "What?!", I of course said yes. He wanted to ask me when I was least expecting it, and he succeeded. Prior to asking me for my hand in marriage, he asked all of my kids for their permission and called my dad for his blessing. Don was still recovering from pneumonia at the time, so couldn't ask my dad in person as he had initially planned.

Per the kids, Don's plan was initially to ask me months later than he did, but this plan kept getting bumped sooner and sooner because he decided he didn't want to wait (and he didn't want me to accidentally find the ring in the house). So, he recruited the kids to help him come up with a plan for the proposal, all while he still wasn't feeling well.

He asked me when all the kids were present at home, including my oldest son and his girlfriend, and it was absolutely perfect for us.

Next, we needed to figure out when and where we were going to get married. Initially we planned to have the wedding in about a year. We started working on finding a venue, and then of the venues that seemed somewhat interesting, we started looking at possible dates. We had trouble finding locations that we both liked or could afford. I wasn't sure when I'd be back to work yet so our budget was very tight, but we believed I'd be back to work sooner than later when we started the planning process, and even still the venues were so expensive.

My youngest son asked why we were waiting, since we knew we were going to get married, and we already felt like a family. We looked at each other and decided that he was right, and we really didn't need to wait, so we could certainly open our search to something in the fall or late summer. We still struggled finding venues but kept discussing places that were important to us as a couple or as a family.

We already had a cruise planned for our family vacation. The cruise we took the year prior was both our first cruise and the first vacation we took as a family, so that gave our cruise this year added importance. We decided to check into whether it was an option to add the wedding on to the cruise, and it was! To our astonishment, the cost of a cruise wedding package was significantly less than even just the location of something local, so we decided to go for it.

The other significant benefit was that there was little planning required on our part. The wedding planners provided us with a packet of information and all we really needed to decide on was which music we preferred from their limited options, which vows we preferred from the options provided, and if we wanted any additional ceremonies within the wedding itself. We weren't planning to invite many people and essentially just wanted a small ceremony with our kids. It all seemed perfectly simple, exactly what my injured brain needed.

While I was excited for the wedding, the cruise itself was making me nervous. All my life I have struggled with motion sickness - I regularly emptied the contents of my stomach in the backseat of cars as I was growing up, or after having gone on too many spinny rides at the county fairs. On our previous cruise, I used anti-nausea patches and anti-nausea wristbands to calm my stomach.

This time around, I was worried about the combination of my motion sickness and vestibular/autonomic symptoms (the balance issues most specifically) I was now experiencing since the accident. I was afraid I was going to have to spend a lot of time away from everyone and miss out on things on the cruise.

Still, it was really nice having something positive to look forward to. As everything else in my life seemed to be falling apart, my relationship with Don seemed to be stronger than ever. We supported each other, never letting a day go by without letting each other know how much we loved and appreciated each other. We were going through all of this together, from the moment of the accident on.

Once I finally started opening up to him about my symptoms and emotions, he shared his feelings about all of it with me, also. The simplicity of wedding planning was brilliant. It was so nice not having to make many plans or really do much for the wedding, yet there was this beautiful thing to look forward to.

The summer went by slowly but quickly. I felt like I blinked my eyes and it was cruise time. The morning of the trip on the way to the airport, we had a car nearly hit us going through an intersection. That scared both of us, and I was crying again in the passenger seat. The stress of getting everyone through the airport, security, getting all the bags checked in, and finding the rest of our group kicked in my dysautonomia symptoms, most notably the enteric nervous system response. I had to make frequent trips to the restroom with an upset stomach. Around these trips to the restroom, I had severe head and neck pain and couldn't focus on any conversations. This was all just while we waited to board the plane.

I booked 7 tickets for our family, but for some reason my oldest son and his girlfriend didn't have assigned seats as the plane had been overbooked, so I was extremely stressed about what was going to happen. We had a shuttle reserved to take us the rest of the way to our final destination, so the thought of us all not landing at the same time made me nervous. About five minutes before we were to board the plane, our entire family finally had seats assigned, but I still was on edge. After landing, getting through baggage claim and shuttling to our hotel, I couldn't 'people' anymore, so we ordered food delivery to the hotel and stayed in our rooms.

The morning of the cruise, Don and I had to get to the courthouse to get our marriage license and then meet everyone at the pier to get on the ship. We had more snafus waiting for transportation and getting everyone to the pier on time, but then we finally had some time to sit and relax once we were all checked in and had been paraded through the pier lobby as part of our VIP status for the cruise.

The wedding itself went swimmingly - there was no stress or drama, just a beautiful, small, perfect wedding. We had our "honeymoon dinner" that night (part of the wedding package) separate from the rest of our traveling party, at a steakhouse on the ship. After a busy day, I couldn't comprehend the menu to order my food and had to have the waitress read me the options and explain them to me. This was a humbling experience and made me very anxious. Thankfully, the food was really good; the company was even better.

Every day on the trip I took naps back in the room. I would go be with family for a while, then take a break back in the room, and go back with family again especially for mealtimes. Even when we went to the beach off the ship on excursion days, I still took a nap under the beach umbrella (because why not?) and rested in the room when we got back on the ship. The kids had a lot of freedom on the ship, and they all did fantastic. They participated in activities and tried new things. I tried being present as much as I could, but as I feared, I missed out on a lot of activities. I would get exhausted and overwhelmed from all of the people, all the activity, all the lights and sounds and smells, and the quiet of our room was absolutely welcomed.

Even still, four days into the trip I started being able to tolerate being out of the room with people less and less. I started to only go out for activities or food, then head back to the room relatively quickly, and I started getting really irritable. We had an appointment to go through our wedding photos and photo packages with the photographer. He took so many beautiful pictures and presented them as an amazing wedding book, but we couldn't afford them because of me still not being back to work and still not getting the disability checks regularly.

We whittled down all the pictures to only a handful of images and bought the rights to these select images to take home with us. I left the appointment in tears because I had to walk away from so many beautiful pictures. I would never be able to replicate those nor the book they had put together and it was emotionally stressful. Looking back, that's probably when I "hit my wall" the hardest. We later found out that our friend who came on the trip had caught a lot of the same pictures as the photographer, in the lounge where the wedding occurred, at least - but we still couldn't recreate the outside photos.

By dinner the final night of the cruise, I could barely stay at the table with the family. I was completely overwhelmed, couldn't converse with anyone at the table and couldn't participate in any more activities. I missed a lot of activities with the family that day. At dinner, the dining room was too loud and there was way too much visual stimulation. My family requested that the speakers near our table be turned down as the music was too loud, and thankfully the request was granted.

I still struggled to remain at the table. I had to switch spots with someone else, so I was facing the wall - facing the whole dining room was too stimulating. Shortly after we were seated, the staff in the dining room prepared for their musical presentation - you literally get dinner and a show at various times throughout the dining times. I couldn't stay in the room during this, however. I had to leave and find a quiet area of the ship until my new husband came to get me and let me know that the entertainment was over. I had been trying to fight back tears as I stood in a back hallway away from the dining and shopping areas. The rest of our group went off to after dinner activities while Don and I went back to the room so I could get some quiet and rest.

The next day was debarking day - which means we got off the ship. We had to catch a shuttle to our hotel, and I still couldn't 'people'. We ordered food to the rooms for lunch and had a quiet afternoon just relaxing and playing cards. I struggled to follow the directions on how to play a card game, but my family was very patient with me. We walked to a local restaurant for dinner and thankfully there was no one else in the restaurant but our family. I was thankful for the relative quiet in the restaurant.

The last morning of our trip was an early one, shuttling to the airport for an early morning flight back home. I was grateful for the quiet of my own home and had to take a nap once we got there. I couldn't even help get the luggage in the house - I needed rest. It took me a week to recover from the trip. I was still overwhelmed, I had severe headaches and severe fatigue. I couldn't do any of my PT or OT exercises due to my headaches and couldn't go for walks. I had simple needs: rest, my bed, my blankets, quiet, darkness. It was a miserable way to spend my second week as a married woman.

14

Lost in resourcelessness

In all the years I've worked in the hospital, we always had care coordinators and social workers that would help patients find the resources they needed prior to leaving the hospital, whether it was helping them apply for state health insurance, finding a primary doctor to see after discharge, figuring out how to obtain their medications, or how to connect with community resources…whatever they needed, there was a team to help them. I was always grateful for this as a provider because I knew my patients would have what they needed to continue healing after leaving our care.

In my time working in clinics and being seen as a patient in clinics in the past, I'm keenly aware that ambulatory (outpatient) settings don't tend to have those same resources. Clinics have nurses that can make some phone calls if you need prior authorization for tests or procedures, but they don't have access to all the community resources you may need, and there's no one helping you fill out all the paperwork.

Clinic staff might get applications to the provider to sign their portion of it, but no one helps the patient complete the paperwork or applications directly. This is left solely to the patient, and often no one asks if the patient needs or has help to complete these. It's not done maliciously, there are just so many requests on a regular basis and so many patients coming through the doors that the staff just do not have the time to do this with every patient.

Now, dealing with this brain injury, there is no social worker or care coordinator for me to reach out to at the clinic to help me. There are only billing and records departments and scheduling specialists that can fax or electronically submit paperwork requested from my providers, but there is no one to help make sure I have done all the things I needed to do. There is no one helping me manage all of my appointments. There is no one helping me connect with the insurance companies to make sure all the documents are sent where they need to go, when they need to go there. There is no one to help make sure I have completed all the documents correctly. It's on me to remember to do all of the things and to do them correctly - me, the one with the brain injury.

Don asked me multiple times if I needed his help, but he was already taking on so much extra work that I didn't feel like I could ask him to do anything else. So, I tried to do it all on my own, poorly, and craptastically failing all the while. I didn't correctly tell the clinic where the bills needed to go, which led to confusion on our auto insurance side of things. I didn't follow up on applications and this led to denial of my long-term disability because I didn't know to follow up to make sure all the documents got submitted correctly. I didn't realize I had to do monthly check-ins with my mortgage lender to tell them I was still off of work to continue my forbearance status, and this almost got canceled. I'm not sure if they never told me about this requirement or if I didn't remember it. Either way, I was making mistakes left and right and didn't even realize it. I didn't know what I didn't know.

Bear with me while I explain this next one. Four years ago, I gave a presentation at the Minnesota State Brain Injury Alliance/Stroke Association annual conference. It had been a bucket list item for me, to present at a statewide conference. I put together a really cool presentation on brain injury (more specifically concussions) and strokes and how they affected each other. I even recycled that presentation and recorded it for my podcast last year. Somehow, I managed to forget about this organization - I forgot they existed, I forgot they were here to help patients and their families after brain injury or stroke...and at long last I finally thought of reaching out to them 5 months after the accident.

On the 4-year anniversary since my presentation (I remembered only because it came up in my memories on social media) I received a packet of information from the Brain Injury Alliance (BIA) with some of the resources they offer. Mind you, these were all in the form of pamphlets and articles - all of which I had difficulty with due to the work it required to see and comprehend what I was reading. I showed all the pamphlets to Don and suggested he would need to help me understand those.

A few days later I received a phone call from the BIA representative assigned to my county. He asked me about all of the therapies I'm receiving, if I needed resources for other therapies, and provided me with contacts for financial assistance, foreclosure protection programs, and support groups. It was such a helpful call. I wish I had made it sooner.

I learned from this phone call that I could have been referred to the BIA from one of the healthcare facilities I had been to, but this hadn't been done. I'm not sure if the facilities also weren't aware of the resources from this organization, or if they just didn't have it in their protocol to share this resource. Had I been referred right away, I would have had access to someone to help make sure I had all the resources I needed, which likely would have reduced a lot of my stress!

I learned that there is actually a social worker available through the county, but there are long wait lists to get help from this particular office. I was aware of one TBI outpatient program in the metro area but learned that there are three big TBI outpatient programs. These are the only programs in the state, however. So, this means that people living outside the metro area still don't have easy access to these programs. I also learned that there are vocational programs through the state to help with job retraining and procurement. I thought these vocational programs were only for people on unemployment, but there is also assistance for people with disabilities, such as brain injury.

Once I identified that I wasn't remembering things well, I tried writing myself notes. I tried very hard to keep track of everything, but I forget things so quickly that if I didn't get something written down right away, it slipped my mind before I could get it on any lists. It was extremely frustrating when I could remember that there was something I wanted to write down but couldn't remember what it was that I wanted to write down.

Many months in, I started a spreadsheet where I logged all of my appointments, all of my messages sent or received to and from my care team, all phone calls to and from the insurance companies, etc., to keep track of what I was doing and when. That way when I didn't hear back from someone, I knew how long it had been since I reached out and could follow up.

I was trying to be more intentional about having conversations with Don. He felt left out of a lot of what was happening. If I had a conversation with a someone about the struggles I was having, I often forgot who I had talked to about it and wrongly assumed that I had told Don, so there were many times that I didn't tell him about phone calls or appointments, and when I would make comments about them later on, he had no idea what I was talking about. This led to arguments because he thought I was keeping information from him intentionally.

He had been regularly asking me what he could help with, but since he was working full time and picking up side jobs to try to make ends meet, I didn't feel like I could ask him to do anything extra. I didn't want to stress him out more about frustrations with the insurance companies, either. And a part of me just didn't like asking anyone else for help. I had always been so independent and never wanted to burden anyone else with things I should be able to do. The problem was, my brain wasn't allowing me to do the things I normally would be able to do, and I wasn't even aware of it. I didn't just stink at multitasking; I was awful at tasking...period.

By opening up to him, I was allowing him to feel more helpful and feel more useful. He was able to check in with me on things to make sure I was getting things done. I no longer took this as a sign that I wasn't doing things well - I knew that he was just helping me. He felt more included, and I'm sure this helped decrease his stress a little because he knew where we were at with applications and bills and everything. The arguments started decreasing because we were a team again.

With savings running dry and no checks from long term disability or auto insurance in sight, we had no idea where the money was going to come from to pay all of our bills. I was able to get a forbearance on the mortgage and one of my school loans for 6 months, but my other school loan could only be reduced slightly for a short period of time, and the rest of the bills remained the same.

Don used to do construction and had his own business, so he still had a lot of his tools and still had the knowledge needed to pick up side jobs building decks and doing odd handyman jobs, but this took him away from the home even more than his long hours at his regular full-time job. The tradeoff was difficult for me as I really needed him present to help out at home. I struggled emotionally with how much time he had to spend outside the house with me not being back to baseline.

I borrowed money from one of my sisters to help cover bills one week when money was not coming in and was careful to pay it back right away when an insurance check came. I did not want to be in debt to people. I reached out to another sister who works with a food pantry, and she got approval to give us a "blessing box", which ended up being multiple carts' worth of groceries and household supplies. I was overwhelmed with emotion at the sight of all of this and cried thankful tears that evening. The kids had so much fun going through all the snacks - it was like Christmas for them.

All the medical bills ran through the auto insurance until that ran dry. Then I called the billing offices for all of the various locations where I was getting care and applied for financial assistance to help pay these bills. I was incredibly surprised how quickly one was approved and overwhelmed at how much personal information others required before the requests could even begin to be processed. When you're a patient in multiple systems with frequent appointments, the bills add up quickly and get to be downright scary.

I have worked multiple jobs over the years and had retirement packages through them all but had lost some of them during my last divorce, so I wasn't sure what I had left. I called one of the companies I knew I still had an account with and was pleasantly surprised that I had a good amount from one of my recent employers. The representative was extremely helpful and talked me through taking a withdrawal on my retirement account. Since this was from a previous employer, there was no hardship evaluation required (or even possible, as I would later learn, because I no longer worked for the company).

The retirement company would take out the taxes and the rep was able to give me an estimate on the penalties that will be assessed at tax time so I would know what to anticipate for that. Taking this withdrawal allowed us to continue paying the mortgage and not lose the house, while I worked on continuing to get better. This was a huge weight lifted for both me and Don, as the financial aspect of me being off of work was causing significant stress for both of us. It was not an easy decision to take funds from my retirement, as this potentially takes away from our future, but I came to the conclusion that if we don't get through the 'now', there will be no future to worry about.

As far as the home front went, I had to ask more of the children. They had their weekend chore lists, but the chore lists got longer. We discussed with the kids that they need to help with their chores during the week, too, not just on the weekends. Earlier in the year we had agreed on an allowance for the kids so they could start learning to manage their money, and this was expected to be their spending money for the cruise. A month before the cruise, however, we discussed with the kids that allowance payments would need to go on a pause because money was getting tight - but they were still expected to do the chores. They were receptive to this and not one of them complained - this was most impressive for a couple of teenagers and a pre-teen.

We preemptively discussed with the kids that I will need even more help whenever I do get back to work. I'll be exhausted from my time at work and will not be able to do as much cooking or cleaning as I even do right now because of it. I expect to routinely hit walls once I'm using my brain daily. Don started a routine of having family meetings periodically to discuss where we are and what the expectations are of family members at the current time. This gives us an opportunity to get input from the kids and help them understand the importance of their roles in the house. It also helped to set a good standard for expectations when school started again in the fall, and I was still in the process of healing.

In general, I've had to swallow my pride and ask for help. I've never been one to ask for help for as long as I can remember. It has been 23 years since I borrowed more than $20 from anyone in my family. With my previous marital and dating relationships, I assumed responsibility for most of the household duties - partly because it was expected of me and partly because my exes then got used to me doing everything and I unwittingly became a bit of a martyr. I learned to not ask for help because I often didn't get it anyway.

It took some therapy after my last divorce to realize that this wasn't healthy behavior and I had to do a lot of work on me before I could take on another relationship. That doesn't mean I learned to ask for help well. I accepted help and was getting better at asking for help prior to the accident, but I still wasn't perfect.

Since the accident, I have felt like a failure in basically every aspect of life because I haven't been able to contribute like I used to, financially, physically, or emotionally, and I didn't want to ask for even more help than my family was already having to offer. By being honest about my limitations and asking for assistance, though, I'm keeping my family in the loop on my needs and how they can help me heal. They have all stepped up amazingly. Who knew that when you let your people in, you grow closer?

I had to learn this same lesson with friends. I didn't want to be a burden on my friends, and this was mostly emotional. I didn't want to lay my troubles on them; I didn't want to show them my weaknesses. I'm always open to having my friends tell me about their concerns and provide support to them, but I didn't want to have to emotionally vomit on them, so to speak. It's amazing how much opening up to my friends relieved some of my stress, and I learned which friends would be the most supportive at the times I needed them. Sometimes I needed to cuss and complain and sometimes I needed prayer and encouragement, and these times required calls or texts to different friends. They were all completely needed, and I love and appreciate them all for their roles in my recovery.

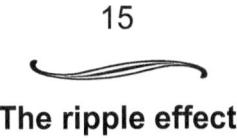

15

The ripple effect

When I used to work in the hospital and clinic with stroke patients, I always stressed to the patients and their families how much they all needed each other. I often reminded them that the patient was not my only 'patient'...the spouses and children were part of the global 'patient' I was responsible for. This was because it's not just the person who has the stroke who is affected by the stroke. Everyone in the family is affected.

If the patient was young, this meant financial concerns and household concerns because the person who was now disabled was still working and contributing to the household in ways that the rest of the family would have to pick up the slack for. This is no different with a traumatic brain injury. I was not the only one affected - my whole family was.

Don carried a lot of blame on himself because he was the driver of the car. He felt responsible for me not being able to work and for us to be tight on money because I wasn't able to work. His full-time job had increased reliance on him because of regular changes at work and them being short staffed, so he was working long hours but wasn't getting any additional compensation because he was a salaried employee.

Because I couldn't work, he was picking up side jobs during the first several months to bring in extra cash, which meant he was working extra weekends and evenings to get these side projects done. This was adding physical and emotional stress on him. He also had emotional stress due to worrying about me and my recovery, as he watched me spiral down mentally and in general not improve physically for so long. He saw small improvements in me, but I never felt they were significant because they weren't getting me closer to returning to work. I was not an easy person to live with.

Because I knew he blamed himself so much for the accident, this was another reason I erred on the side of not telling him how bad I was for so long. I didn't want him to blame himself even more than he already did. I thought I would improve much more quickly and that it would just be better if I kept some of this to myself. The problem with this was that he then didn't know the severity of my symptoms. Once I realized I was struggling, I didn't tell him I was struggling because I didn't want him to worry, but that backfired because problems would arise, and he was unaware of them. In the end, keeping my symptoms from him only made things worse.

He didn't want to use any medical money from our auto insurance for his own issues because I needed so much medical care. This meant he didn't get evaluated for his constant headache that was likely related to a concussion, as well. He also didn't get evaluated for back and shoulder pain that likely also were accident related. He had injuries many years ago that hadn't bothered him also in many years, but suddenly were bothering him again after the accident, unfortunately to a much more severe pain level. He put off care to minimize his own need for medical bills to focus more on my recovery. There was no amount of encouragement that was going to change his mind on this.

I couldn't be fully present with my kids. Yes, I was able to attend some activities with them for school that I may not have been able to had I been working full time, but I didn't feel really present. I always had a headache, so I spent a lot of time on the couch with my head covered. The kids could be in the same room as me, but they needed to be quiet. I couldn't interact as much as I would have liked because of my headache and my inability to remember things well.

I didn't want them to be bored all summer, so I occasionally tried taking them to parks, the lake, thrift shops - anything that was free or cheap, but we could only go for a little while because I would hit my wall and have to leave, go home, and take a nap. I felt bad for cutting things short so often. I started getting easily irritated with the kids. I was raising my voice more often than I'd like to admit and had a lot less patience when they were just being…kids.

I have been a dog person all my life, but after the accident I wasn't a good dog mom. I couldn't take the dogs for walks because my balance was off and the Labrador, specifically, is a tank and she would easily be able to knock me off my balance and I would potentially fall over. I would forget whether the dogs had been fed or not. Initially they started gaining weight because they were actually getting fed too often, then they started sitting by their bowls because I would forget to feed them.

I got irritable with the dogs, too. I would push them away when they would try to get attention or leave them outside longer than I normally would because I just didn't want them next to me. One of the dogs started having behavior issues and began going to the bathroom in the house. We believe this was because she wasn't getting attention from me, and her favorite person (Don) wasn't home as much due to all his extra work. The dogs did not like this new arrangement.

I decided to ask my family members for their direct feedback, to get their take on what was happening. When I asked my husband, Don, he admitted that he didn't understand things at first. It seemed like I just didn't want to go to work, and he didn't understand that because he'd never seen me like that. A few months in, he physically saw me hit my wall and saw my entire demeanor change - my facial expression, everything; I just seemed "checked out". That's when he realized there was something more than just me not wanting to get back to work. He wished he would have realized sooner how serious my symptoms were.

When my mood became an issue, he wanted to help, but knew all he could really do was just be there for me. Sometimes it seemed like I was trying to push him away because I kept asking him if he was sure if he still wanted to marry me and then after the wedding I kept asking if he was sure he didn't regret marrying me; I was concerned because of my brain not working and me being angrier all the time. He did feel some stress because I was leaning on him for all of my adult interaction, since I wasn't going to work and wasn't spending much time with other people. He felt pulled in all directions, trying to work and get his schoolwork done, spending time with the family, and trying to have some down time for himself.

His role had to change from just being partner/spouse to caregiver, which affected our intimacy to some degree. He was exhausted from all the extra work he was doing, and then we were arguing more; both of those factors would decrease the desire for intimacy. It took some work to remind himself that he needed to think about my needs and desires and not just his.

Don struggled a lot watching me not notice my own improvements. He would see little wins but would get frustrated when I didn't see them. He tried to point these out to me, and he always got excited when I was able to notice them and got excited about the wins myself. It took him almost 9 months to step in and help me manage my healthcare, and he wished he would have done it sooner. He kept thinking it would get better, but when things weren't getting better, he decided to get more involved.

Then there's the guilt Don felt. He was the driver and went through a red light, yet I took the brunt of the injury in the accident. He wished he would have been alone, or the accident would have turned out differently because he feels responsible for me not being able to work and provide for the family like I used to. He admitted the feelings of guilt were huge. He also wished he would have been around more to help me initially and admitted that work was a bit of an escape for him. He knew he needed to provide for the family, so he took that literally and put everything into his work. I asked him multiple times to spend more time at home and said I needed him, but he didn't understand that for so long, and he felt bad that he listened but didn't hear.

When I asked the children for their feedback, my adult child, Shawn, wasn't quite as affected (because he had his own place with his girlfriend and didn't see the daily struggles). The biggest thing that he noticed, therefore, was that first, I was unable to help them pack up and move when they moved 4 hours away for his girlfriend's schooling. I have been involved with all of his/their moves, but I was not available for this one because that was right after the accident and my symptoms were too severe.

162

The other way he was affected was on our family vacation. I had to take frequent breaks back to the room and couldn't tolerate a lot of time with the family, so I didn't get to spend much time with them on our trip. For example, I was excited to watch them play in a pickleball tournament, as I'd never actually seen anyone play it before. I messed up the time they were playing and missed the tournament completely. They ended up taking second place in the tournament, which I was both excited and saddened to hear - it would have been so much fun to watch them earn this.

My middle child, Hayden, noted he couldn't do things as much with me like we used to, like going for walks. He also felt like my injury took away from him being able to have real conversations with me because he was afraid of how I would respond. He stated he couldn't predict how I would react and was often afraid I would get upset at things, though I never actually did. He felt worried about emotional responses that didn't actually happen, just because he couldn't read me.

When I started a new therapy around the 6-month mark that was finally helping me turn the corner toward improvement, he was the first to call out my improvement by saying, "Welcome back", hence the title of this book. He no longer worries about my responses and feels like I'm more back to normal compared to prior to starting my new therapies, thankfully. He feels like I'm making near constant improvement.

My youngest child, Bryce's, first response was "you were less happy". He didn't like that I couldn't help him with as many things as normal and I couldn't go on as many walks as we usually did. He felt sad because he "couldn't do as much stuff" because I couldn't do as much stuff...well said, kiddo. He was scared when he first found out I had been in an accident because he didn't know what was going to happen to me, so he was really glad to see me when he came back from that weekend at his dad's house.

When we started getting really tight financially, he loaned me $20 to help with whatever we needed help with. I tried telling him that he didn't need to loan me money, but that was sweet of him to offer. He wouldn't take no for an answer, and said if I needed more, he would loan me more. He's good at saving his allowance money, unlike his siblings. He also noted that I always seemed more tired and less able to respond when things were happening in the house, and he admits this happened a lot when the kids were doing things they weren't supposed to. He was really excited to tell me he could see a HUGE difference when I finally started improving.

When I asked my step (bonus) daughter, Becca, about how she felt affected by my accident, she described it as a chain reaction. She noted that we have a house full of empaths, so when she noticed more stress with me or her dad, it caused stress with the boys and her, and ultimately everyone felt the stress. She was nervous for the transition to a new school, specifically going into high school, so this all just added to her stress with the transition.

She said that even though we tried not to show the kids our stress, she could feel it. She noticed when Don and I were arguing more because we generally didn't argue. But she also saw me trying to focus on the positive things, which helped her also try to look for the positives in her life and not focus on all the negatives.

All of this is just anecdotal evidence from my own home that I was not the only 'patient'. My whole family was affected by my brain injury. I was constantly amazed by how my children (biological and non) have been able to learn my triggers and how to help me. They have been incredibly supportive when I have tried to do new things, when I tried on various occasions to get back into regular physical exercise, and when my PTSD got triggered when we were in the car. They adapted to me needing to take breaks and they would ask *me* how I was doing.

I was equally amazed at my supportive partner in all of this and his ability to identify when I would hit my wall before I noticed, as well as his gentleness when I just needed to be held and allowed to cry because everything was all so overwhelming. I couldn't have asked for a better squad of humans to call my own in this journey.

16

Finding God in the journey

I have struggled with my faith for years, having gone through 2 previous unhealthy marriages and rough divorces, and following the last divorce being diagnosed with at least one autoimmune disease, which took away some of my physical abilities. My youngest child had behavior issues which took us away from going to church, and while I felt something was missing in my life, I found it hard to go back. I would have conversations with friends or family about my struggles and they would recommend prayer and keeping faith, but I felt like my faith was lost. I would "check out" when they would continue talking and shut down, and they could see it.

Finally, after reaching out to my sister and getting the blessing box, I didn't shut down when I had 3 friends talk to me about needing faith and prayer in my life. The series of events over the next couple of weeks was nothing short of miracles. We held a garage sale to raise money. We had things to get rid of and needed the extra money, so we made it happen a week after deciding to do it. One of my friends came over to help set up and made quick work of preparation for the sale. During the sale, we had several people give us larger bills to pay for their purchases and tell us to keep the change. That never happens; people usually try to barter to pay less for things at a garage sale, not say "keep the change".

I didn't have to argue or fight to get money out of my retirement account, and the company rep was extremely nice and helpful in the process. The first application I completed for financial assistance with one of my medical providers was quickly approved the first time applying. I received cards with money from family members who were on a fixed budget that I would never have asked for money from, with notes of encouragement in the cards. I have no explanation for all of these things happening other than 'Thank you God'.

Then came the biggest gift I could have asked for. As I previously mentioned, my boss would check in with me regularly for updates and to share anything she had learned about new treatments that may be helpful for me. This time she wanted to tell me that one of our surgeons started up a new clinic for alternative treatments to help people heal from athletic and neurological illness, including TBI, and she wanted me to connect with him about it. I have looked into every option she recommended, and unfortunately wasn't able to act on most of them because they were out of pocket expenses, and we had empty pockets.

I was always open to information about new therapies, though, so I spoke with the surgeon about this new option. He shared some great reports from the patients they had already treated and wanted me to come in for treatment. The biggest gift: he didn't want me to worry about the financials - he just wanted me to get better so I could get back on the team. I was nearly in tears on the phone, and just like when they had offered me the job to work with them, this was an offer I couldn't refuse (nor did I want to!).

17

The breakthrough

During our phone call, the surgeon noted that a year prior he wasn't aware of all of the alternative treatments that he now knew about, and he had become passionate about offering these treatments to his surgical patients to help them heal faster after surgery, and he was astonished at the improvements seen with other patients who had suffered from traumatic brain injuries. He did note that their injuries were not to the same extent as mine, so he didn't want me to think it would be a miracle overnight cure.

He noted that I had been doing all the right things, all the typical things we recommend for patients with TBI, but that I was just a prisoner to time and these alternative therapies could help me get better faster. In fact, my neurologist had recently told me it was time to look 'outside the box' because we had tried everything 'inside the box' and nothing was doing the trick. Here was my 'outside the box' opportunity.

The surgeon explained that he wanted me to come in three times a week and eventually try out all the variety of therapies they had to offer at the clinic. The protocol he would have me start on was the same as prescribed for NFL players when they sustain TBIs, to get them back on the field faster. I needed to get back to my team, and he believed this would help.

When I got to the clinic that first day, I learned about the variety of therapies offered, including a couple forms of laser treatments, red light therapy, structured water, pulsed electromagnetic frequency (PEMF) mat, and exercise with oxygen therapy (EWOT). All of these therapies were proven to help the brain heal faster after injury, and some were even being used to treat post-covid brain fog and being researched to help people with Alzheimer's dementia. So much research has been done. I wasn't ready to read it, but it was fascinating knowing it was there.

My first treatment included breathing misted structured water while sitting on the PEMF mat, followed by transcranial laser therapy, as well as direct class IV laser to my low back. I have a history of back injuries, but this pain had also been significantly increased after the accident, likely from the jarring impact of the vehicles. Before I even left my first appointment, I had reduction in my headache and neck and back pain as well as improvement in my thinking. Throughout the day I noticed less word finding difficulties, better mood, and I was able to converse with my family (and call a couple of friends to tell them about the appointment) and not stumble over my words or slur. I had so much more energy and was talking nonstop - I had six months of not talking much to make up for!

The clinic where I do these new treatments is called HyperCharge Clinic™, and I literally felt like I was having my brain jump started, which led to another drawing.

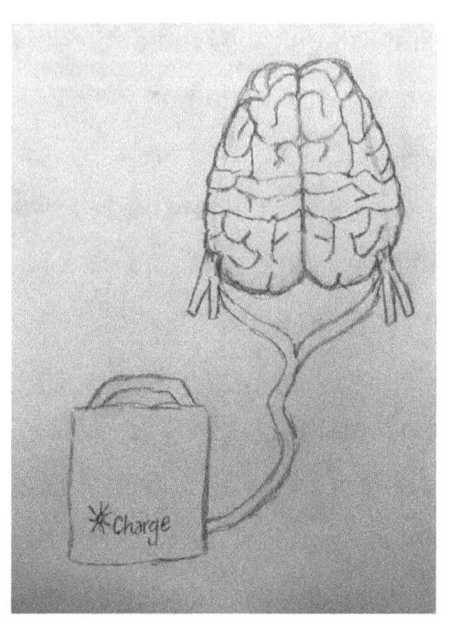

I drove my middle child to swim practice the night after my first treatment, and I talked to him nonstop there and back. He finally looked at me with a goofy grin on his face and said, "Welcome back". His response nearly made me cry.

The next day, I woke up with a massive headache (which I now know is a Herxheimer response - increased pain 24 hours after treatment), but I was not going to let it get me down because I had been warned it wasn't a miracle overnight fix. I remained hopeful for the cumulative effect. This was new to me. I forgot what it felt like to feel hopeful and to be excited for the healing process. I had been so focused on the fact that I was not making any real progress for the last six months that it became very difficult to see the minimal progress I was making. Now I had taken a huge jump. Yes, the headache was back, but I was otherwise nothing like I had been the day prior to starting these new therapies.

I went back for the second treatment and again had a reduction in my headache. I felt another boost in my energy. I had multiple appointments later that day, including PT and OT and I was able to attend them all without hitting my wall. Testing identified improvements at PT and OT for the first time in months. I was able to do tasks for both of them and not need a break in between. Both of my therapists noted a shift in my mood, and I was so glad to tell them I finally felt hopeful. Just because I was seeing improvement finally didn't mean therapies would end - the new treatments would just augment what I was working on with PT and OT.

The next day, I went to lunch with a friend. As I told her about the events of the week, she said

"Welcome back" (this seemed to be a growing theme) and I didn't hit my wall while we ate and talked at the restaurant. That evening I recorded my first podcast in 6 months - as the interviewee. One of my best friends is a mindset coach. She had been encouraging me to find some way to share my story with people.

I was at the point that I had no more pre-recorded podcast episodes to launch and would need new material, and for the first time in 6 months, I felt like talking. So, I invited my bestie to interview me on my show and we discussed a plan for a series of interviews to share my story on the podcast - the accident, the road to recovery, the hiccups I learned about - all of the things that would ultimately be laid out in this book, as well. This bestie and another good friend both had been encouraging me to share my story in book format when I was ready. It took a long time to feel ready, and a lot of work to even start putting things down in any kind of semblance of organization.

In the first week of these new treatments, I met with my mental health provider and again had to do my regular screenings for depression and anxiety. Both scores had a significant reduction. She was energized by my huge shift in mood. She was getting ready to take a couple of weeks off for vacation, so my improvement was perfect timing for her, she said, as she was concerned about me not having support for two weeks.

Though I was nervous to record a podcast episode again and was literally shaking like a leaf during the recording, the finished product was inspiring. My best friend and interviewer told me "Welcome back" because I finally sounded more like myself again. Listening to the recording, I heard what she heard, and this gave me the confidence I needed to keep at it. I reached out to organizations that would be good to feature on the podcast to focus on concussion and TBI for the next season of the show. I reached out to some of my providers that I wanted to highlight. And my heart swelled with pride when I got positive responses. I finally felt a little more like myself.

A week after starting the new treatments, Don and I went to dinner, and he pulled into the parking lot of one of the stores we used to walk around. He was excited that I was feeling better and hadn't hit my wall yet and wanted to take me there to walk around because "we could". It was so nice to do this simple yet remarkable thing together again. I was not feeling back to 100% yet, but I was significantly better. I was so much better than I had been the day prior to starting these new treatments.

Little by little, I noticed I was requiring less use of my prism glasses (especially the computer glasses - these seemed almost more problematic now), I was experiencing less intense headaches, had less irritability and more energy. I was getting more talkative and was doing more laughing and more smiling.

That said, there continued to be areas where there was no improvement. I noticed no improvement in my peripheral vision yet and I still couldn't go completely without my prisms. The headache reduced in severity, but a mild headache still remained always. I still felt some slips with word finding, but nothing like what it was, and it didn't seem to be noted by others as much as I could feel it myself. I still couldn't remember everything, but my memory did feel a little better at least.

I still struggled with reading comprehension, but found I had the ability to do a little bit of reading and some of the words made more sense than they had been (this isn't saying much, though, since it was *such* a struggle for so long). I read many positive remarks from others who had had similar treatments. I briefly clicked around on the websites for the new technology and found that some had been featured on other podcasts and they had research posted on their websites that showed treatment efficacy. I still couldn't comprehend the research articles, but it was promising to see that there has been research done to support these treatments.

In the second week of treatment, we added additional treatments, including whole-body red-light therapy and exercise with oxygen therapy (EWOT). My exercise tolerance tanked after the accident because of my autonomic symptoms, so I couldn't do the exercise on the stationary bike, but instead used a vibration plate in place of the "exercise". The first day using the vibration plate wiped me out. I needed naps again during the next couple days. For the second day with the vibration plate, we decreased the total time on it to hopefully prevent the fatigue and return of the required naps.

After a week of vibration plate and red light, I was more fatigued and more irritable. I was not sleeping as well at night and still needing more naps. At the end of the week, I was knocked out with a whopper of a headache. My PTSD symptoms were again getting triggered by any little mention of an accident or by seeing an emergency vehicle on the road while we drove.

After going a week without needing my noise canceling earbuds all the time, I needed them more than ever and needed to be back under my blanket in a dark, quiet room. I felt like it was a huge step backward. I checked in with the clinic and learned I was having a 'healing crisis'. Adding all the different treatments had me essentially 'drinking from a firehose' and we needed to back off to a garden hose again. This was a little disheartening, but I tried to keep an open mind.

The next week we would be removing the vibration plate and red light and go back to the basics with the structured water, PEMF, and transcranial laser. After one day of this reduced treatment protocol, I was not quite as fatigued and the headache seemed a little better again, but my memory was still delayed compared to the previous week and I was still irritable. I still chose to stay positive, which again is something I hadn't been able to do for 6 months.

I was reminded that it was a miracle I wasn't in pieces due to the impact of the accident, and any improvement I was experiencing now was more than I had prior to starting these treatments. I felt blessed to have the improvements I was seeing, and I looked forward to continuing to improve and hopefully getting back to being me again. Well, me 2.0 - hopefully I come out of this a better version than I was prior to the accident.

I'm learning firsthand that healing is not linear. I kept saying throughout the process that I wish I had just broken a bone. With a broken bone, you get a cast, you maybe have surgery depending on the severity, but you have a deadline for healing. You will heal and you can almost mark the date on the calendar (barring any complications). You don't get that luxury with brain healing.

My injury took me from my baseline and dropped the floor out from underneath me. That process was quick and relatively linear - I just dropped. However, the road back is more like the game *Chutes and Ladders* - you may come to a square in the sidewalk where you hit a slide and fall backward, or by some miracle you hit a square that has a ladder and you get to rise up quickly...but beware, there are other squares with slides again. And there's rain and bad weather along the way, and the road is unnecessarily curvy.

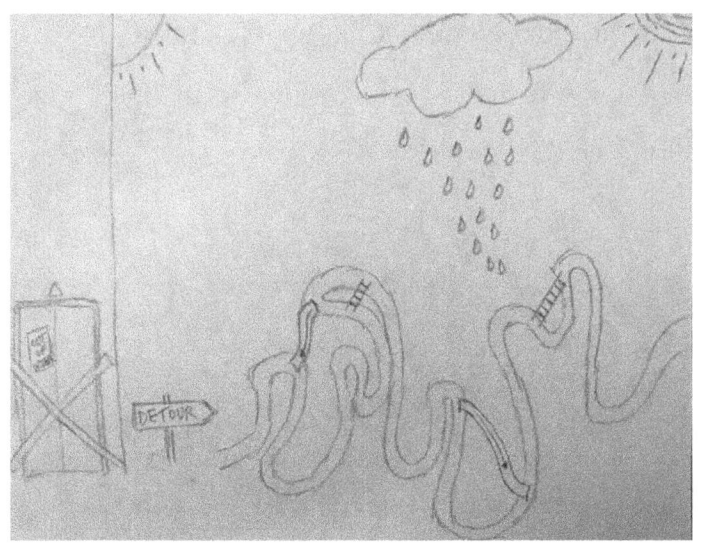

There are ups and downs in the healing process, and you have to come to terms with that, so you don't spiral down mentally anytime there's a step back. Two steps forward and one step back is still one step forward, after all. And I was no longer taking baby steps to get better - the pace had picked up slightly, so we'll call them toddler steps. There were still stumbles and still tears, and the improvement wasn't as fast as taking nice big adult steps forward.

As frustrating as it is, the ups and downs are part of the process. I have always hated the phrase 'trust the process' - it implies that things will not go smoothly but you need to keep faith. I hate the phrase because it's true. It's the 'not going smoothly' part that gets me every time.

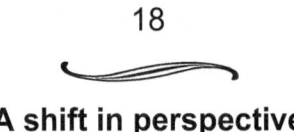

18

A shift in perspective

I had many people tell me I needed to change my mindset. For so many months I struggled seeing the positives in anything - the minimal improvements I was having didn't seem substantial to me, and they certainly didn't get me any closer to getting back to work. Everyone told me I just needed to change my perspective, I needed to be thankful for the improvements that were there, I needed to focus on the positive because focusing on the negative all the time wasn't helping me. You think? I knew I needed to change my mindset. I knew I needed to focus on the positive. But at the moment all I could come up with was "I'm positive this sucks" or "I'm positive I'm not getting better fast enough" and I would give a half-hearted smirk.

It was considerably easier said than done to just change my mindset. I had run out of hope. I didn't know what hope felt like anymore. I didn't see a light at the end of the tunnel - there was just darkness everywhere. I wasn't me anymore. I didn't feel like a nurse practitioner. I didn't feel like a productive member of my family. How in the world was I supposed to see positives when there weren't really any positives to see?

The day I started the new therapies with the cranial laser and all that jazz - that's when my mindset changed, the first time. One single appointment and treatment improved my mood, my energy level, my speaking, my headache…one single treatment gave me hope. My hope was back. My motivation was back. And even though there were still setbacks, I knew they wouldn't be permanent. I knew in the grand scheme of things I was still improving. The cumulative effect of continued treatments and continued therapy would bring me continued improvement, and I could finally see that. So, while the improvement wasn't as fast as I had hoped, it was still improvement, and there was no going back to what I was prior to starting the new therapies.

I can try to put into words what that new perspective meant to me, but I don't think I can ever do it justice. I needed hope with my entire being. I needed the light at the end of the tunnel. I needed to feel like I hadn't lost myself. I had been going through the grieving process of losing my identity, so I needed something that could let me know that my identity wasn't lost. And here I was, finally, feeling hope again.

19

Surfacing symptoms

Once improvements started in some areas, it became evident that I'm the human, less-appetizing version of a parfait...I have layers. When the laser treatments reduced my headaches, I could feel all the other pains in my body more from the accident, more specifically the back and neck pain. When the dizziness was improving, I could more clearly describe the problems I was having with my vision. As my word finding difficulties improved, I was better able to describe my cognitive difficulties. More than 7 months into recovery and I was just starting to be able to describe some of my limitations. What a frustrating scenario, to think you're finally starting to improve only to realize you have more layers that need help.

This is the point where speech therapy started, to work on my cognitive deficits. Having worked in neurosciences for as long as I have and having close friends who are speech therapists (more correctly, speech and language pathologists or SLP), you would think I would have known that speech therapy worked to improve cognitive deficits, but you would be wrong. I had no idea. In the hospital, I always saw the OTs doing the cognitive evaluations, so I assumed this fell under the OT category. At my initial SLP eval, however, I learned that it is actually SLP that works on cognitive deficits, so she was to become my new best friend.

Because I was essentially no longer struggling with word finding or stuttering with speech, I started having people make comments like, "I'm surprised you're not back to work yet because you seem fine". You've got to love the invisible disability of brain injury. The few physical scars I had left on my arm from the airbag were now hidden by long sleeves thanks to the cold midwestern weather, so I had no physical limitations left that others could see. For the most part, I could carry on conversations fairly well if we were talking about the kids or mundane daily things. And for the most part, if we were one-on-one, I could converse for a decent amount of time. But that's all most people would see.

What they didn't see while we were having those conversations is that I would get distracted if something else was happening in the room. If we were in a room full of people, I still couldn't follow conversations well, and I likely wouldn't remember much of any single conversation at that point. Therefore, I still usually avoided social situations that involved a lot of people. This and I would still get overstimulated, and my headache and dizziness would kick in, even if I had my noise canceling earbuds in. I had to leave my best friend's birthday party early because of this.

I also skipped Thanksgiving with my larger family because I knew I would still get overwhelmed in the house with multiple people. The last family gathering we had in the fall had great weather and I spent most of the day outside away from the large crowd of people - that's the only way I could stay as long as we did.

191

What people also likely didn't notice in the mundane day-to-day conversations is that I still couldn't access my medical knowledge. Eight months into recovery and I still did not feel like a nurse practitioner. I found some game apps on my phone for medical quizzes and thought maybe they would help spark my memory. Nope, I just failed miserably. I tried to look up journal articles to read and couldn't make it past a few sentences before my brain turned to mush and I couldn't understand what I was reading. Same with my review books I have at home. I felt like I was trying to read something in a foreign language. I tried to watch short continuing education programs I found online and couldn't stay focused long enough to complete them.

I became more aware of these lingering deficits than ever because of the improvements I saw in other areas. I've had conversations with others through podcast interviews to find that I'm not the only person who has experienced this, either. It's actually quite common for people to find improvement in some of their symptoms only to realize other problems that they perhaps weren't quite aware of prior or didn't seem like as big of an issue. So, it appears brain injury recovery is kind of like peeling back the layers of an onion - you remove one layer only to find yet another layer that will sting and make you cry.

20

The rollercoaster

The next few months felt like a rollercoaster of emotions - and I've never been a rollercoaster fan. I stayed on my high from the initial improvements after starting the red light and laser therapies for a couple of months. I loved the new energy and the sense of hope. But I was frustrated by the lack of improvements in cognition. At the 9-month mark, I graduated from PT because my balance had improved significantly and was now only an issue when I hit my wall. I remained limited by autonomic symptoms when the wall was hit, however, including my balance being off.

When I started with SLP, I also transitioned locations for OT and started more aggressive therapy for my continued visual difficulties and comprehension related to my visual impairments. We began so many new exercises, and I literally started seeing improvements (pun intended). We experimented with different colored protective sheets to put on the computer screen to have less eye strain. We progressively increased the difficulty levels on exercises where I first identified just the letters on a chart, then had to come up with a word that started with that letter, and then had to try doing the exercises with background noise. I did graduate from prism glasses...briefly...and a month later had to put the prisms back in the glasses again. My eyes weren't quite ready for that leap.

With SLP, we did more cognitive testing, and I was extremely disappointed to find that my visual comprehension remained at the first percentile, meaning 99% of people who took the tests I did scored higher than me. I have beyond a master's degree yet still couldn't comprehend well what I was reading.

I added two more mental health therapists to the list of appointments. In addition to my individual therapist, we now had a couple's therapist because we were feeling a lot of strain on our relationship. She has been amazing at helping us both work at eliminating traumas we both have from previous relationships that were now starting to cause issues with our fragile new marriage, as if my anger issues alone weren't enough.

I also added another therapist who was certified in EMDR (eye movement desensitization and reprocessing) to work on the PTSD. I still wasn't getting any better with driving, and the question was raised if some of my cognitive issues were also related to the PTSD. After effectively creating a mental "safe space", we started digging into the feelings surrounding the accident and reframing my thoughts about the accident itself. Two months later, I was able to drive through "the intersection" and see emergency vehicles on the road with no more reaction than I had prior to the accident. This felt like a freaking miracle. But it wasn't quite letting my cognition improve yet.

I finally got word that long term disability was being denied again because of my history of migraines. I was so angry I couldn't even create a response right away. I reached out to my last two employers and asked them to write me letters spelling out that I had missed very little work in the last 2.5 years prior to the accident, and in fact worked above a full-time status the entire time. My neurologist also wrote a letter stating that my lack of ability to return to work was due to cognitive deficits, not headaches. So, I wrote up yet another appeal letter and sent it off…I'm still waiting on a response.

The lost wages through auto insurance were tapped out around the 9-month mark, also, so I literally had no income to help offset any of our bills. I opted to take another withdrawal from retirement because there seemed to be no other option. I had applied for financial assistance through the county, the state, and local offices, but we were just over the cutoff for a family of five. Essentially the only expense they considered was mortgage, not school loans, vehicle loans, or the extremely expensive utility bills to keep our home running, much less any other expenses we have with 3 children still living at home.

I started having darker feelings again because of my inability to get back to work and my subsequent nonexistent income. My EMDR therapist had a handy book of therapeutic things to talk about - I jest but this book was really full of good information! During one of my sessions, after I had repeated for the umteenth time that I just wanted to be able to think like I did prior to the accident, we talked about acceptance. She shared an excerpt from her therapy book that described the relationship between pain and acceptance:

Pain + nonacceptance = suffering
Pain + acceptance = pain

She described this as pain (whether physical or mental) when combined with nonacceptance (meaning you don't accept your current circumstances) leads to suffering. That same pain when combined with acceptance (accepting your current circumstances, but you don't have to like them) leads to pain only; the suffering part is optional. I giggled (as I tend to do when I inappropriately deal with everything through humor), not because of the words, but because of what it reminded me of...the path to the dark side (for any Star Wars fans out there):

> *Fear, leads to*
> *Hate, which leads to*
> *Anger, which leads to*
> *Suffering, which leads to*
> *The Dark side*

So now my goal was to avoid the dark side. I needed this conversation so much. I was so dead set against accepting anything less than what I had prior to the accident that I wasn't allowing myself to see the gains I was experiencing.

I felt like I was stuck in permanent patient mode - being a patient was now my full-time job. I was able to do my podcast a little more efficiently again, so there was one win, but it wasn't enough for my confidence. Finally, one day while I was getting my red light and laser treatments done, the founder, who was the primary practitioner treating me and now also a friend of mine, once again dropped a hint/joke about me working with them. I stopped and asked if that was a legitimate offer, and a couple more conversations and only 24 hours later, I was hired and had a start date. I would start doing the laser treatments that I had now been receiving for 4 months. I decided this was something I should be able to do because I had been a client for so long and all I would need to really learn was how to run the machines, and I could use "cheat sheets" for that.

There was much more than how to run the machines to learn, and I was very overwhelmed when I started orientation, but it felt good to be doing something other than being a perpetual patient. It was a long way from being a nurse practitioner, but it was something, and the team I got to work with was phenomenal, and super understanding of my limitations. I was humbled and grateful.

I started working only two days a week for 3 hours at a time. I was tired when I was done, and I started hitting my wall regularly again. The plan was to increase my days and hours, and ultimately my responsibilities at the clinic while my brain was

201

healing. I would work these hours around all of my appointments. I kept doing my own therapies at the clinic 3 days a week, as well as my weekly OT, SLP and mental health appointments. I continued following up with my neurologist and neuro-optometrist (eye doctor). My primary care provider was now in the mix as well, as I finally admitted defeat with my mood and needed to start on medication to help me.

We made changes to my red-light bed protocol when newer technology became available, and the new settings on the bed gave me more energy. I was finally able to start adding the exercise with oxygen therapy at the clinic, on the bike, and even exercise on my own at home. Until I started working, I was able to exercise regularly. Once I started working, however, I was back to the same balancing act I had previously with my therapy exercises vs regular exercise. If I got in all my days at work, I couldn't get in all my exercise. I could only spend so much energy in a day.

At the 11-month mark, I gave my first presentation since the accident. In my series of TBI-related interviews on the podcast, I had a guest from the Minnesota Brain Injury Alliance come on the show to talk about the resources available to TBI survivors in Minnesota (all states have BIA offices, but not all states have the same resources), and following that interview, I was asked to speak at the spring conference for TBI survivors and share my story of going from provider to patient. I was incredibly nervous to give a presentation again, though I've been in front of audiences for decades. Ultimately, I thought that if I was going to stumble over words during a presentation, what better place to do it than in front of a bunch of people like me - brain injury survivors? I hit my wall hard after that presentation, but it was so worth it.

The process of putting together my speech was almost therapy in itself. I became more accepting of my current circumstances and came to some realizations. The hospital may not be the environment I return to whenever I get back to being a nurse practitioner, but I will do something rewarding. After starting to work even a handful of hours every week and spending the time that I did to prepare my presentation, I started noticing something else - my brain was starting to make connections. Occasionally, I would blurt out something medical related to a situation, and I would think to myself, "Where the heck did that come from??" (but it usually wasn't heck that was said in my head...or even out loud).

My speech started becoming more fluid - even the people at work noticed this. I was no longer pausing in my sentences to think of the next word. I started remembering the settings on the machines. I started being able to read bullet points in the manuals and taking notes. By the way, I was taking notes on everything! I hand wrote notes on everything I was learning at the clinic and would review my notes daily. I started being able to look up things related to neuroanatomy, taking notes and drawing pictures to locate different parts of the brain or spine. Hope was returning.

So, here I am, almost exactly 1 year since the accident as I write this paragraph, still not back to being a nurse practitioner, still struggling to feel useful on a regular basis, still struggling to feel like myself, but I'm seeing the improvements I've waited for so long to see. I still have good and bad days. On my good days, it's easier to identify how much improvement there has actually been and it's easier to stay hopeful. On my bad days, everything still triggers me, and I occasionally retreat to a dark place where hope does not exist. These bad days happen more after I've done something that made me hit my wall hard, or times when our bank account reminds me that I need to get better faster.

I hit my wall more frequently because I'm testing my limits more often, but as long as I take a break and rest, it doesn't take me as long to recover. I'm still limited by time due to autonomic symptoms. If I push past the 3-hour mark and try for 4 hours or more, I hit the wall. If I try to do this two days in a row, I'm toast. When I hit my wall, I still get tired, I start becoming unsteady and off-balance, I start slurring my words or stumbling over words or not being able to complete thoughts well, I get a severe headache, and apparently, I can't park my vehicle very straight. I'm waiting on an appointment with a provider that specializes in dysautonomia to hopefully get further information on this hurdle.

I'm still working with all of my therapists and am extremely grateful for the whole team. And it's still hard for my family to watch, yet they remain my biggest cheerleaders.

This week, I went for my first run...well ok, jog. I went 2.5 miles, and it was amazing. About the 2-mile mark I started feeling dizzy and off-balance, so I took it easy since I still had to get home. My next goal is 3 miles without symptoms.

21

From voice to paper

You may wonder just how in the world I was able to write a book given my cognitive troubles. Short answer is it was a process and I had help. Longer answer is it was a longer process than I expected, and I had help where I least expected it.

At first, I couldn't write sentences, but I could make bullet points. That made it easy to lay everything out in some sort of organization. When I was able to think more in sentences, I slowly turned the bullet points into sentences and put the sentences together. Then I took it in chunks and read through it, often out loud when I was home alone, to see how it sounded. I utilized the spell check feature (and grammar) because I was in no shape to spell or use grammar correctly. This sounds funny coming out of my mouth because I was spelling bee champion three years in a row in grade school, and I've never had a problem spelling anything...until this recovery process.

As I would read through sections, I would think of something I wanted to make sure I talked about and quickly find a way to add it. Then I would read further into the chapter and find I already included it...ugh...time to go back and delete everything I had just written, because I didn't need to say it twice.

Through all of my podcast interviews, it has been a common theme from folks I interviewed who wrote books that writing was a form of therapy. It helped them mentally and emotionally move forward after writing about their experiences. Some of them never intended to publish but were encouraged to by others, and then they were glad they did. In all instances, though, the writer gained so much from the experience.

After running into snags and hurdles in my recovery process, I was determined to share my experience to hopefully help others. That is what I've done all my life, so why would I stop now? I've always said when I have a medical issue that God was just teaching me empathy to be a better provider. I could have used a smaller lesson with this one, in my opinion, but I've definitely learned things in this process that I will take back to practice with me, whenever I get there.

I have a newfound drive to ensure that future patients who experience concussion and more severe TBI get the care they deserve and don't have to fight so hard to be treated. I don't know what all of that looks like yet but sharing my story on my podcast and in this book, and sharing the resources I did in the podcast, as well as highlighting other people's experiences with TBI, is a great start. Having one presentation under my belt, I have applied to be a speaker for a couple of other conferences and applied to be listed as an available speaker with a couple of organizations, as well.

I look forward to the day I can get back to my normal line of work and get the ultimate "Welcome back" and have the opportunity to share the lessons I've learned from this experience with my patients directly. One year down, forever to go.

Reference

1. Viswanathan, W., Gu, W., Blanch, R., & Groves, L. (Retrieved 11/21/23). Cataracts after Ophthalmic and Nonophthalmic Trauma Exposure in Service Members, U.S. Armed Forces. *Military Medicine*, usad414, https://doi.org/10.1093/milmed/usad414.

Learn More

If you'd like to learn more about the resources shared on the podcast, please look up Brain Wellness - the Podcast on your favorite podcast listening app. I'll include the URLs for Spotify and Apple Podcasts here:

Spotify: https://spotifyanchor-web.app.link/e/S7kS4ap5Eub
Apple: https://podcasts.apple.com/us/podcast/brain-wellness-the-podcast/id1651330166

If you'd like to learn more about my previous book on migraines and how to contact me (including all the social medias), this biolink will take you wherever you want to find me: https://bio.link/brainwellnessnp

About the Author

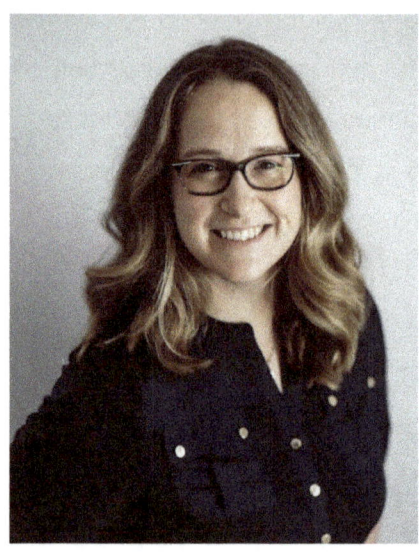

Mandi Dickey is a Board-Certified Nurse Practitioner with 20+ years of experience in healthcare. She is a three-time *Top Nurse Practitioner* award winner, received the *Faculty Excellence* award in her previous role of nursing professor, has been on the review committee for several nursing textbooks, and was the recipient of the *Women of Armor Personal Growth* award for 2023. In 2022, Mandi began her own podcast called *Brain Wellness – the Podcast*, covering a multitude of topics related to brain health and wellness, and has been interviewed on multiple other podcasts, discussing migraine and stroke treatment and concussion prevention.

In 2023, Mandi was in a car accident and suffered a traumatic brain injury, and while not fully recovered, has returned to her passion of sharing and educating the public about neuroscience topics, now most passionately about concussion and TBI.

d

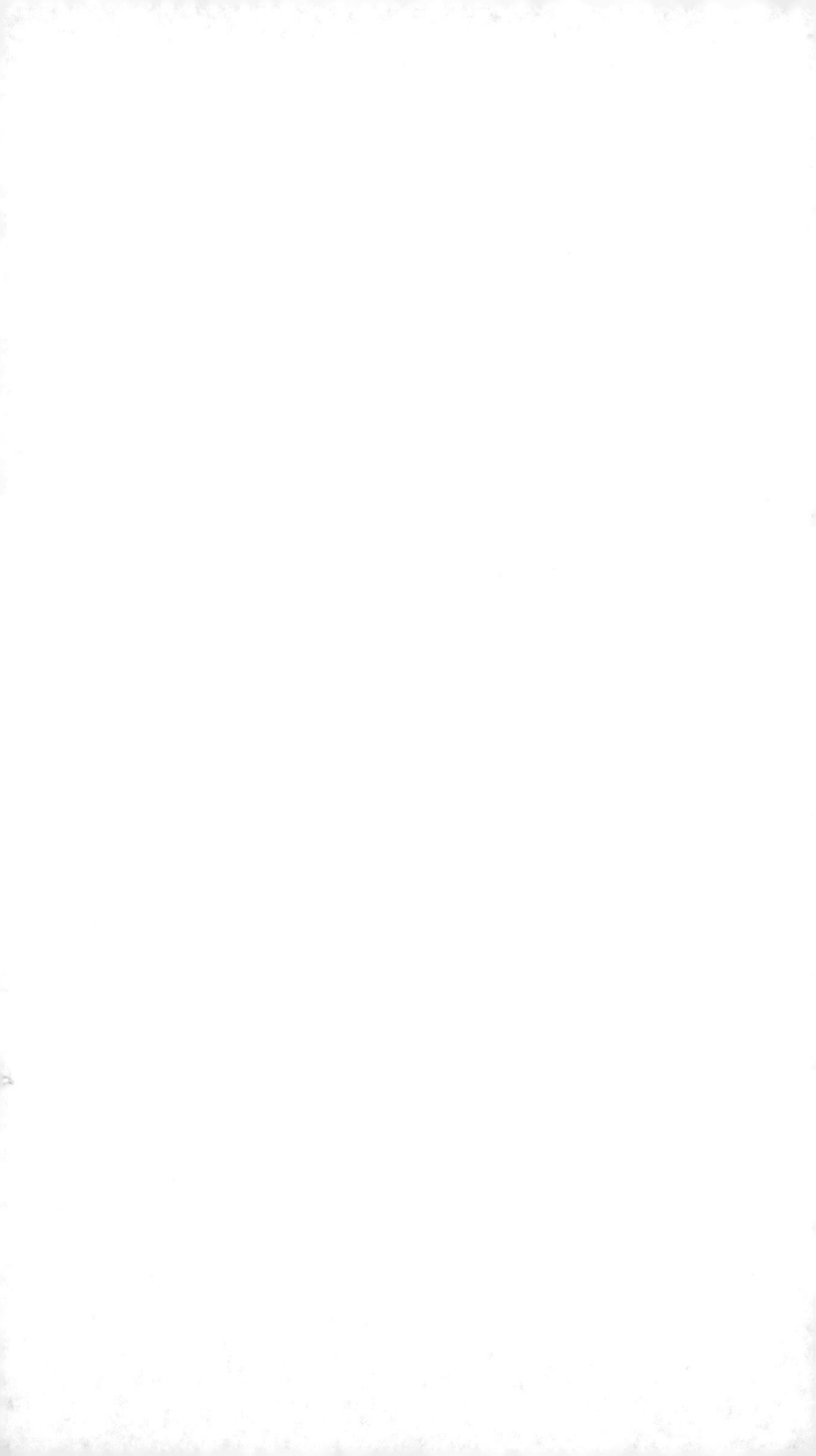

www.ingramcontent.com/pod-product-compliance
Lightning Source LLC
Chambersburg PA
CBHW060502130626
46553CB00002B/392